PERCEIVING CRUCIAL SYMPTOMS

S.M. Gunavante

B. JAIN PUBLISHERS PVT. LTD.

Reprint Edition 1996

© All rights reserved

Price : **Rs. 25.00**

Published by :
B. Jain Publishers Pvt. Ltd.
1921, Street No. 10th, Chuna Mandi,
Paharganj, New Delhi - 110 055 (INDIA)

Printed in India by :
J.J. Offset Printers
Kishan Kunj, Delhi - 110 092

ISBN 81-7021-408-4
BOOK CODE B-3958

Dedicated to

DR. S.P. KOPPIKAR, *who, during 14 years of his Editorship of "The Homoeopathic Heritage", scooped out, month after month, the gold mine of invaluable advice with case illustrations from the pioneers and other able practitioners - and thus provided immense inspiration and unequalled guidance to the upcoming generations in the science and art of Homoeopathy;*

and to

DR. RAJAN SANKARAN *who has been focussing a flood of light on many of the gray (neglected and insufficiently grasped) aspects of homoeopathy through lectures, video cassettes and writings (especially his book "Spirit of Homoeopathy"), and is helping homoeopaths towards fulfilment of the ideals envisioned by Hahnemann.*

Preface

There is a considerable amount of literature about the comparative value of symptoms and how to apply that knowledge in practice. However, the subject is really deep and complicated; and different masters have laid varying emphasis on different classes of symptoms. As a result the student gets quite confused. It is for this reason, probably, that Dr. Elizabeth Hubbard wrote:

> "In science and indeed in any art... the greatest and simplest truth must not only be reiterated but constantly presented in striking and varied lights so as to evoke from other minds new channels of thought and new vistas for investigation".

This guideline is my apology for presenting this work.

We shall, therefore, view the entire landscape from Hahnemann down to Rajan Sankaran and focus attention on the most crucial symptoms which can guide us easily and quickly in the accurate selection of the remedy in a given case. I have particularly in mind four crucial methods for selecting the simillimum.

Firstly, the unique importance of perceiving the "state of mind and disposition" as stressed by Hahnemann in Aphorisms 210-213 of the "Organon". The usefulness of this approach has been so ably illustrated by Dr. Rajan Sankaran through case after case in his book, "The Spirit of Homoeopathy". Every Homoeopath should cultivate this art and experience for himself the thrills of its success in practice.

Secondly, the classical "Totality" which takes into account the uncommon, peculiar symptoms of Mind, Physical Generals and Peculiar particulars, including the symptoms of the Active dominant miasm.

Thirdly, in those cases where the approaches just mentioned are not feasible (because patients are not frank, or unobservant or are heavily compensated in their shocks, disappointments, etc.) the Homoeopath will find it necessary to depend on the peculiar symptoms combined with Physical Generals. How such cases can be tackled is also shown in one Section in this book.

Fourthly, the importance of investigating into the Chronic (latent) infections and identifying the Nosode called for has been examined in detail in another Section. This much neglected aspect calls for more than casual attention.

Fifthly, there is a method of selecting the remedy - the celebrated "three - legged stool" approach of Hering; also known as the "Minimum Syndrome of the Maximum Value" as advocated by Sir John Wier, Candegabe, Mrgaret Tyler, etc. This approach has been explained in my book "Gennius of Homoeopathic Remedies".

In order to fully understannd those approaches, it is essential to study Hahnnemann's instructions in the Organon. Essential points on the most important of these Aphorisms have been given in Appendix 'C'

The way in which Hahnemann's instructions have been interpreted and applied in practice by his disciples such as Boenninghausen, Lippe, Boger, Allen, Guernsey, Kent, Margaret Tyler, including the latest contribution of Dr. Rajan Sankaran, have been examined in detail in the relevant Sections.

The potency problem insofar as it is a component of the Perfect Simillimum, including the question of the repetition of the dose in the management of the case, has been briefly dealt with.

The book concludes with a Section on "Conclusions and Plan for Action". It is hoped that the book will be found to be a useful and practical guide in the effective practice of Homoeopathy.

Moraya Villa
12th Road, Khar,
Bombay 400052.   S.M. Gunavante
Tel. 649 8146
1st November, 1993

CONTANTS

	Preface iv	
1.	Introduction. 9	
2.	Compilation of M.M. and the Organon. 11	
3.	Changing perceptions of Symptomatology. 14	
4.	Boenninghausen's Totality. 17	
5.	Dr. C.M.Boger's approach to Case Analysis. 22	
6.	Totality according to Dr. H.A. Roberts. 27	
7.	Peculiar, characteristic symptoms and keynotes.- Guernsey etc. 29	
8.	Perceive the most uncommon (unusual) Peculiar Symptom. 40	
9.	Take positive symptoms irrespective of the "drug picture". 42	
10.	Totality of symptoms. 44	
11.	Contribution of Dr. J.T. Kent to the advancement of Homoeopathy. 46	
12.	Kent's Repertory - how to use it. 52	
13.	What to do when strong mentals are not available. 57	
14.	Why are particulars less important in remedy selection? 62	
15.	State of disposition and mind chiefly determines selection. 65	

16. Dr. M.L. Sehgal's "Rediscovery of Homoeopathy"........ 82
17. State of body - Effects of latent (chronic) 89
    Infections (Miasms). - Understanding the Miasms - Psora, the hydraheaded Infections - Meeting the challenge - Tracing the link between the Infection and the remedy -Tyler on Nosodes - Stop-spot of Remedies - Symptoms of leading Nosodes - Illustrative cases.
18. Remedy response - Second prescription - Management of the case. 123
19. Conclusions and Plan for Action 133
20. The Best Test of a Homoeopath. 147
    Appendix 'A' - Physical Generals. 149
    Appendix 'B' - Peculiar Symptoms. 153
    Appendix 'C' - Important Aphorisms from the Organon. 154

1 Introduction

The practice of Homoeopathy needs a thorough knowledge of this system of therapeutics both as a science and an art. The scientific aspect covers the philosophical view it takes of health, disease and the principles of curing the deviations from health. However, mere knowledge of these principles is not sufficient for putting them into practice. One has to acquire the technique of putting the principles into practice, including the art of dealing with unexpected problems, which comes only through actual practice. Expertise in any branch of knowledge or line of activity comes only from practice, just as one can learn swimming or cycling or driving a car only by actually getting down to action - involving the risks of temporary failure and setback before one masters the art of success.

To be a successful practitioner of Homoeopathy, one must

(i) master the principles and philosophy of this science directly from the pen of masters, such as the "Organon of Medicine" (Hahnemann), Genius of Homoeopathy (Stuart Close), Principles and Art of Cure by Homoeopathy (H.A. Roberts), Lectures on Philosophy (J.T.Kent), etc.

(ii) learn the technique of taking the case and understanding the patient.

(iii) master the principles governing the evaluation of symptoms elicted from the patient in order to be able to pick out those which are of crucial importance in selecting the remedy. One has to develop this ability under the direct supervision of an able practitioner.

(iv) learn the essential, characteristic and individualising features of remedies in the materia medica-we may call them the GENIUS of remedies - so as to be able to compare the crucial symptoms of the patient with those of the remedies, and select that remedy which bears the closest resemblance to the patient under treatment.

(v) administer the remedy in the proper potency and repetition, and manage the case through ups and downs following requisite measures such as hygiene, diet, repetition of dose, etc. as may be necessary, till the patient is fully restored to health.

In this five-fold study of homoeopathy as outlined above, we are concerned, in this book, only with step (iii), viz. learning the art of identifying the symptoms of crucial importance in a case as guides in the selection of the similimum. Nevertheless, a brief reference will be made to the other steps, as a background study for step (iii).

2 | Compilation of the Materia Medica and the "Organon".

Once Hahnemann was convinced about the law of cure. viz. that a medicinal substance which is capable of producing symptoms in a healthy person can cure similar symptoms found in a sick person: Like cures like, or "Similia Similibus Curentur", he took the next logical step of finding out the symptoms which various drugs could bring forth, in healthy persons. This was called "Proving" of the drugs. If the drugs had not been proved, we would not have known the peculiar and characteristic symptoms of each remedy, since such symptoms alone have to be matched with the peculiar and individualising symptoms of the patient. The "proving" symptoms thus form the indispensable basis for selecting the remedy.

During his lifetime Hahnemann proved almost 100 drugs with the help of his family members, friends and others. His close, meticulous supervision of the provings, combined with his clinical experience with those medicines, gave him the unique insights into the various problems which arise in the practical application of the Law of Similars. His observations on the working of this law and his clear guidance regarding the principles which should govern the application of the law have been laid down in the "Organon of Medicine".

"Organon" our Guide : For mastering the priciples of homoeopathy, one cannot do better than study the instructions laid down by Hahnemann in the "Organon of Medicine"

"Organon" our Guide : For mastering the priciples are homoeopathy, one cannot do better than study the instructions laid down by Hahnemann in the "Organon", especially on what is disease, the vital, force and the symptoms that should guide in the selection of the curative remedy. The relative Aphorisms are given, as succinctly as possible in Appendix "A". Hahnemann revised the "Organon" five times after vast experimentation, close observation and deep reflection. The Organon today is a high water-mark in medical literature, providing an indispensable source of guidance in solving all types of problems confronting a prctitioner. The books by Stuart Close, H.A. Roberts and Kent are a clear elucidation of the principles.

The reader is advised to go through Appendix 'C' from time to time, as by doing so the importance of the philosophy which must guide practice will form part of your mental make-up. This will also enable you to understand and grasp the true significance of the elucidation given by the various pioneers on various aspects of symptomatology and other related matters.

(ii) **Taking the case :** Hahnemann has laid down instructions to guide the practitioner in eliciting the required information about each case of disease. The examination and interrogation of the patient in order to obtain the type of data pertaining to the mind, body and suffering of the patient is unique for homoeopathy and is different from the examination undertaken by the modern school. These instructions are given in Aph. 83 to 144. Further elucidation of this important task is given by Dr. Pierre Schmidt (The Art of Interrogation). Bender (The Examination of the Patient). and Dr. Rajan Sankaran (Spirit of Homoeopathy).

(iii) Study of Symptomatology follows in the next Section.

(iv) **Genius of Remedies - our working Tool :-** Knowing as we do the vast symptomatology of each of the remedies in the Materia Medica and the difficulty of remembering the numerous symptoms in detail, with consequent inability to recall them readily, an attempt has been made by us to present the Genius of about 90 of the most commonly used remedies in a separate book "The Genius of Homoeopathic Remedies." Each remedy has been divided into eight clearly defined class of symptoms. Without such a handy and concise yet dependable **Working Tool,** the prescriber faces an uphill task in locating the remedy whose characteristics closely match those of the patient. It is hoped this "Genius" will considerably lighten the task of the prescriber in selecting the simillimum.

(v) **Management :** The questions of potency, repetition of dose and of management of the case are dealt with briefly in Section 18.

3 Changing Perceptions of Symptomatology

We observe from the Aphorisms in the "Organon" that Hahnemann has repeatedly stressed the "totality of symptoms" as of prime importance. At the same time, he strongly affirms in Aph. 153, that "the peculiar, uncommon, singular, striking, (characteristic) signs and symptoms are to be chiefly and almost solely to be kept in view". Even while stating emphatically that the "state of the disposition often chiefly determines the selection of the remedy" (Aph.211), he advises us in (Aph.213) to select a medicine which "in addition to the similarity of its *other symptoms* to those of the disease, is also capable of producing a similar state of the disposition and mind". It appears that this dichotomy (of clubbing "other symptoms" with the "state of disposition and mind") has resulted in his followers placing varying stress on "Totality" on one hand and "Mind and disposition" on the other according to their predilection. Further, since symptoms of mind and disposition are very difficult to elicit, even Boenninghausen chose to give only a few Mind symptoms in his "Therapeutic Pocket Book". C.M.Boger, a deep student of Boenninghausen, did not expand the Mind symptoms very much in his "Boger Boenninghausen's Repertory", beyond Boenninghausen's list.

It is true that one of the masters like Boen., Boger, St. Close,Roberts, Kent or Rajan has departed from the perception of "Totality of symptoms" repeatedly emphasised by Hahnemann in the "Organon". Yet a perceptible, though subtle, change can be noticed in the emphasis they place on different class of symptoms. It is necessary for a practitioner to be familiar with all these subtle variations so that he may apply one or the other of them depending upon the prescribing data he is able to elicit from each patient. We shall examine them in detail herebelow.

Dr. J.T. Kent was a stalwart head and shoulder above many others in his mastery of Philosophy, his deep knowledge of Materia Medica as well as in his ability as an artistic prescriber and teacher. As such his contribution in guiding homoeopaths on the path of practising classical Hahnemannian homoeopathy enabling them to deliver the full benefit which the homoeopathic system is capable of giving to ailing humanity, has been massive. We shall go into his teachings in more detail in the relevant section which follows.

While following Kent (and Hahnemann) closely, Dr. Rajan Sankaran has in recent times shown through precept and example (through Video and case illustrations) that Hahnemann's emphasis on the "State of Mind and disposition" of patients (Aph.211-213) is not mere academical. and if properly understood and brought into practice is capable of yielding immense advantage in our efforts to find the true simillimum, with all the benefits to the suffering patients which no other system but Homoeopathy can confer.

The task of finding the simillmum is beset with various difficulties. There is one more way of simplyfying this task, viz. the use of the "three legged stool" of the "Minimum Syndrome of the Maximum Value" approach. This approach is nothing but using a very small group of the most Singular and Characteristic symptoms to identify the remedy, and later to verify its correctness by reference to the "Genius of Remedies", or a more detailed Materia Medica.

These changing perceptions of symptomatology need to be appreciated by the Homoeopaths at large if we are to develop the skill to perceive the CRUCIAL symptom or symptoms which hold and key to any given case.

4 Boenninghausen's Totality

It should be said to the credit of Boenninghausen that in those days of "infancy" of Homoeopathy, he classified the numerous symptoms in the provings/materia medica into five classes : (i) Location of complaint, (ii) Sensations of pain like burning, throbbing, cutting, cold or heat, etc. and, (iii) *Modalities* i.e. conditions of aggravation or amelioration of the complaint. To these he added (iv) *Concomitant* or associated symptoms and (v) *Causation*. His task in making these classifications was difficult in as much as the symptoms recorded by the provers were not complete. He observed that provers gave modalities of one part, and a sensation of another, whereas it was only when one had a **complete** symptom (giving location, sensation and modality together - and possibly causation and concomitant) that it could be usefully taken to form the totality. Therefore, his brilliant, analytical mind resorted to the principle of analogy, by which he concluded that the modality (or sensation) or one part could be taken to be applicable to symptoms of any location or part or even the whole person.

It is on this principle that he constructed the **Therapeutic Pocket Book,** a Repertory for use at the bedside and in the study of the materia medica. About this book Hahnemann wrote in Footnote 109 in the Organon, "Dr. Von Boenninghausen, by the publication of the characteristic symptoms of homoeopathic medicines and his Repertory has rendered a great service to Homoeopathy."

The Therapeutic Pocket Book is divided into seven Sections: (i) Mind and Disposition, about which he wrote: Most beginners in homoeopathy are liable to overlook this part of the picture of the disease or to make mistakes. Therefore, I have considered it wise to give here only what is essential and prominent, under as few rubrics as possible in order to facilitate reference. (ii) The second Section covers " Parts of the Body and Organs". (iii) The third Section contains the Sensations and complaints (a) in general, (b) of the glands, (c) of the bones, and (d) of the skin, (iv) The fourth Section treats of sleep and dreams. (v) The fifth of fevers, (iv) Conditions of Aggravation and Amelioration (vii) The seventh and last section gives "Concordances" in place of the Relationship which was earlier published by him. Boenninghausen says in his preface to the Therapeutic Pocket Book : "From one point of view the Conditions of Aggravation or Amelioration have a far more significant relation to the totality of the case and to its single symptoms that is usually supposed. The correct choice of the suitable remedy depends very often chiefly upon them."

Concomitant symptoms : The discovery of the existence of Concomitant symptoms in many remedies. whose number he was able to expand from his own long experience, led Boenninghausen to place them together under each Section. Boenninghausen's emphasis on the importance of the Concomitant symptoms has led to the statement that his repertory is "founded on the doctrine of concomitants". H.A. Roberts corrects this to say: "the doctrine of the totality of the case, which must include the concomitants". Roberts adds further: "The concomitant symptom is to the Totality what the condition of aggravation or amelioration is to the single symptom - It is the *differentiating factor.*"

Symptoms occur in groups : Boenninghausen

recognised that symptoms naturally occur in groups some of which are marked and prominent and some are subsidiary. In constructing the Pocket Book he proceeded on Hahnemann's theory that it is the man who is sick, and that all his discomforts are a part of his condition, and are therefore to be considered together to bring him to a perfect cure. The human organism is like a great complicated machine, composed of many parts assembled according to a definite plan or idea. The repertory, with its classification of symptoms is like a stockroom of a factory, with the parts stored in a perfect order. The workman selects the parts necessary to form the machine and assembles them according to the plan. According to this plan, the assembling of parts has to be meaningful to give us a working machine. In the same way, the totality is not a haphazard collection of symptoms. They must fit together to portray the picture of the patient as well as the remedy as seen in the materia medica.

Peculiar Symptoms, the basis of Homoeopathic prescription:

Boenninghausen had observed in the course of his extensive practice that symptoms appear in constantly varying combinations in provings as well as in sickness. The form which they take are governed by the peculiarities of the individual. Each case will present certain typical, common, diagnostic symptoms; but they will also present what Hahnemann calls uncommon, peculiar (characteristic) symptoms which represent the individualising factor of the case. These individualising symptoms differentiate one case from other cases. The Hahnemannian doctrine is that these *peculiar, uncommon symptoms* either on the mental or physical plane, really represent that which is curable in each case of disease, and they are therefore the BASIS OF THE HOMOEOPATHIC PRESCRIPTION. It is for these peculiar symptoms that the similar remedy must be found, rather than for those general symptoms which appear commonly in almost every case and almost in every remedy.

A way into the wide field of combinations : Boenninghausen's genius lay in bringing the fragmented parts of symptoms together through his plan of assembling the parts not at random but by seeing that each part has a definite relationship with the others. The totality thus erected reveals both the remedy and the disease. Another practical obstacle he had to face was how he could combine the symptoms, even of the same remedy, if they were experienced by different provers. His answer to this problem lay in his plan of the repertory. It had the avowed object of opening., as he put it "A WAY INTO THE WIDE FIELD OF COMBINATIONS". If two different provers had reported two different symptoms of Lycopodium, it meant that Lyco. has the capacity of producing both of them, therefore they could as well be taken as if they were found in the same sick person. It is this unique insight into the nature of incomplete (fragmentary) symptoms produced by the provers on the one hand, and the equally varying groups of symptoms presented by individual cases on the other, and the need to construct a bridge between such diverse elements, which led Boenninghausen (confirmed by his experience) to present his Plan of the Repertory as a "WAY INTO THE WIDE FIELD OF COMBINATIONS". Without this basic philosophy behind the construction of the Repertory, the immense benefit which we derive today from the Repertories would not have been possible. The advantages of this approach will be appreciated when we contrast it with the rubrics in Knerr's Repertory to Hering's Guiding Symptoms. Knerr has not broken up the symptoms, but has presented a location with a sensation together, or a location with a modality. This system makes it very difficult to apply the rubrics to the ever-varying grouping of symptoms presented by patients.

Rank of Remedies : Another innovation credited to Boenninghausen is the rank he assigned to the remedies in each rubric. He distinguished (evaluated) them principally into four ranks: CAPITALS (4marks), **bold** face (3), *italics* (2) and roman (1). In assigning a higher or lower rank, he says, "No industry, care nor circumspection has been wanting on my part to avoid errors as far as possible". This device for showing the comparative rank of remedies in each rubric continues to guide practitioners to this day.

We have dealt at this length with Boenninghausen's contribution to the construction of the Totality, since a major part of whatever he said continues to be valid.

It is worth pointing out that the Therapeutic Pocket Book has guided homoeopaths for over a century. It has run through many editions and translations. Hempel, Okie, Boger and T.F. Allen among others, have given of their time and genius in attempting to perfect this little work. The latest edition was revised by H.A. Roberts with a detailed, very instructive introduction.

5   Dr. C.M. Boger's Approach to Case Analysis

Dr. Cyrus M. Boger was a close student of Boenninghausen's works and philosophical approach. He had an immense practice with all kinds of illnesses. He has left behind his four important works, viz. "Boger-Boenninghausen's Characteristics and Repertory" "A Synoptic Key of the Materia Medica", and "General Analysis " (being an introduction to Boger's Card Index Repertory) and "Studies in the Philosophy of Healing" A study of these works shows that Boger **generalised** many conditions when they were found in more than three parts or organs. He used pathological generals, such as Bluish, Convulsive, Black (discharges, skin, ulcers), Offensiveness (of discharges, expectoration, leucorrhoea, menses, urine, sweat), Moistness, Yellow, Discharges amel., etc. He regarded them as representing the tendency of the whole constitution.

About generalisation Boger said : "In ordinary practice generalisation is least understood and very often neglected to the detriment of good work. A curative prescription can only be based on "generals" which include and are derived from the "particulars". Generalisation is one of the most important functions to be performed by the prescriber in the process of selection of the curative medicine. It should be further realised that the FINER HOMOEOPATHIC ART demands the perception of the rule that "the highest rank of all belongs to those symptoms that are not only peculiar but are also general."

Boger followed Hahnemann's central idea that "the further a given symptom seems removed from the ordinary course of disease, the greater is its therapeutic value".

In analysing a case, Boger first took the anatomical sphere where in a symptom arises, then the Modalities of aggravation or amelioration of that symptom, and out of the few remedies that would emerge from this process, the mental outlook as given in the pathogenesis will do the final selection. Boger thus was not in favour of opening a case with mentals (as advised by Kent), but with Modalities (general and particular) and Concomitants. He followed Stuart Close's advice in his Genius of Homoeopathy, "Mental symptoms, when they appear in the record of a case, are always of the highest rank as material for *final generalisation and completion of the totality upon which the prescription is* based". In fact, he said: "Although mental symptoms are highly significant and attractive to the choice, correct or incorrect, they are not as dependable as guides against a wrong choice of the remedy as the great physical generals."

While writing about Modalities, Boger observed: "All of these indications are so trustworthy, and have been verified by such manifold experiences, that hardly any others can equal them in rank - to say nothing of surpassing them." In fact, the Synoptic Key opens with Modalities as the first chapter.

The last chapter of the "Characteristics and Repertory" on "Conditions of Aggravation and Amelioration" is extremely useful particularly because it is comprehensive, comparing favourably even with the corresponding chapter on "Generalities" in Kent's Repertory. Roberts says of this chapter, "These often outweigh in importance the known relationships of specific circumstances to specific symptoms. In other words, the general may be more safely trusted than the particular unless the particular denotes both the remedy and the patient."

Boger's Classification of symptoms: Based on his vast experience, Boger evolved a system which depends upon a three-fold classification of symptoms.:

1) The fundamental, constitutional or *life-time effects;*

2) The presenting complaints, which are a *fresh or acute outburst* of the deeper-lying tendencies;

3) *Modalities.*

Hierarchy of Rubrics for case analysis : Boger gives in his synoptic Key the diagram of the hierarchy of rubrics to be followed for analysing a case. One has to follow it in practice to appreciate its advantages.

MODALITIES : Caustion. Time. Temperature. Weather. Open air. Posture. Motion, Eating and drinking. Sleep. If alone. Pressure. Touch. Discharges.

MIND : Irritability. Sadness. Fear. Placidity.

SENSATIONS : Burning. Cramping. Cutting. Bursting. Soreness. Throbbing. Thirst.

OBJECTIVE ASPECT : (Expression of sickness): Facial Expression. Demeanour. Nervous excitability. Restlessness or torpor. State of Secretions (colour, consistency, odour).

Lastly : the PART AFFECTED (Organs, right or left side). This brings the investigation in touch with the diagnosis.

Boger concludes: The above rubrics in the ORDER

NAMED point fairly well towards the simillimum, and the prescriber has only to bear in mind the fact that THE ACTUALL DIFFERENTIATING FACTOR MAY BELONG TO ANY RUBRIC WHATSOEVER.

Dr. S.R. Phatak, who was an excellent prescriber, had found the Synoptic Key to be his most dependable guide. He once told Dr. P. Sankaran that in the course of 25 years he had by constant use completely worn out at least six copies of this book. Dr. Phatak's "Concise Repertory" has drawn much from this book.

The last appearing symptom : Boger describes the last appearing symptom as one of the first importance in the choice of the remedy. "Ranking close behind, or even at times taking precedence of the peculiar and general symptom, must be placed the last appearing symptom of a case". Gibson Miller has stressed this point almost in these same words in his "Comparative Value of Symptoms". Boger illustrates this point in his "General Analysis" through a case of Lichen Planus, in which Rheumatism amel. in damp weather was the latest symptom, which guided to the remedy.

Concomitants : Writing about concomitants Boger says in his Preface to his "Characteristics and Repertory":

In finnding the simillimum for the whole case the Cancomitants above all, demand the most thorough examination... We must, therefore, examine all these accessory symptoms which are:

(i) Rarely found combined with the main affection, hence also infrequent under the same conditions in the provings;

(ii) All those belonging to another sphere of disease than that of the main one;

(iii) Finally, those which bear the distinctive marks of some drug, even if they have never before been noted in the preceding relation.

H.A. Roberts further clarifies the role of concomitants in his Introduction to the "Characteristics and Repertory". He writes, "The totality of the case meant to Boenninghausen (as it no doubt did to Hahnemann) a matter of concomitance - a group of related symptoms not expressing the disease so much as expressing the individual who suffers... It is the totality of the symptoms - the whole picture of the suffering man - that must be considered; and this is made up not alone of the symptoms one expects to find... but those found in other parts of the suffering individual. For example, nausea and vomiting mean little as such, but if they are accompanied by, say, backache, noises in ears, suffocation or tongue clean, we often get a picture that is clearly indicative of the certain indicated remedy, the simillimum. Therefore, concomitance is a sound doctrine of procedure in homoeopathic prescribing for, the more "strange, rare and pecualiar" the symptom grouping is, the more atypical for the disease syndrome - the better guide we have for the selection of the perfectly indicated remedy.

6. Totality According to Dr. H.A. Roberts.

A few observations of Dr. Roberts from his "Principles and Art of Cure by Homoeopathy" will be in order.

The personality, the individuality of the patient, must stand out pre-eminently in the picture... This embraces not only his physical characteristics, but the expression of his mental and emotional characteristics as well.

The generals rank the highest in evaluating the case; without generals we cannot expect to find the simillimum. At the same time, the mental and emotional characteristics have a high value since these are the true reflections of his personality, the man himself.

In fact, the simillimum is practically never found among the diagostic symptoms.

If we allow ourselves to be guided by the symptoms of the patient, (not the diagnosis) which are an infalliable guide, we shall probably save the patient, even though THE REMEDY SELECTED ON THE BASIS OF THE SYMPTOM TOTALITY MAY NEVER HAVE BEEN USED UNDER LIKE DIAGNOSTIC CONDITIONS BEFORE.

The symptoms of LOCATION frequently furnish quite characteristic symptoms.... Certain types of diseases localise in certain parts, like gout in the great toe, and yet are of systemic origin....localisation in the left or right side of the body, or in the base or apices or middle lobe of the lungs; on which side the trouble starts and in which direction the symptoms move and where they localise, as for instances throat troubles going from the left side to the right, or from the right side to the left, or continuous alternation of sides. These are all PECULIAR, characteristic symptoms.

Besides the concomitant symptoms, there may be one in which the GENIUS of the remedy is plainly and definitely portraryed, so that it would be immediately noticeable. This symptom would immediately attain such importance that would OUTWEIGH THE CHIEF AILMENT in chosing the simillimum. Such a symptoms correspond to Hahnemann's dictum about striking, strange, peculiar and unusal symptoms. It may be considered *alone* in choosing the remedy because it gives pre-eminently the character of the whole design.

No medicine can cure any disease unless it acts upon the diseased parts, either directly or indirectly... One organ cannot suffer alone any more than one cell can suffer by itself.

Very often the concomitance of circumstance is of greater importance to the whole case than the expressed sensation.

The character of the drug is represented not by a single effect, but by A GROUP OF EFFECTS. This group is the only representation we have or can have of the medicinal character of a drug . . . . these effects are the only relationship that can be established between the medicinal effects of a drug and the disease.

We must not fail to **recognise** the value of the TOTALITY of the symptoms; and this must take into consideration the chief complaint, those of which the patient most often complains, plus the peculiar characteristics of the patient ... If we can find a remedy that has the "more striking, particular, unusual and peculiar (characteristic) signs and symptoms" of the case and if IN ADDITION it covers the Chief complaint as well, we may consider ourselves as having a sound basis for the prescription of the simillimum.

7 | PECULIAR, CHARACTERISTIC SYMPTOMS AND KEYNOTES

Guernsey, Ad. Lippe, H.C.Allen etc.

Of all the Aphorisms in the Organon the most widely studied, discussed, accepted and practised Aphorism has been the 153rd. The emphasis in it on the "more striking, singular, uncommon and peculiar (characteristic) signs and symptoms of the case which must be chiefly and almost solely kept in view" is unqualified. It has been found to be applicable to any component of the totality, irrespective of whether it is Location, or Sensation, or Modalities, or Concomitants, or the symptoms of Mind and disposition or even the symptoms of parts of body (Particulars as Kent called them). However, the process of identifying these Peculiar, characteristic symptoms from the vast materia medica was not easy. Dr. S.P. Koppikar gives a brief review of this process in the "Editor's introduction" to an article "On Characteristic Symptoms" by Dr. J.H.P. Frost (Hom. Heritage Aug. 1991)

"Between 1850 and 1900 - those years when our materia medica grew wonderfully - every homoeopath had to be a good student and scholar. In trying to find the right remedy from the totality of symptoms of the patient, the problem of the VALUE of the symptoms was the main topic of discussion. Many tried to follow the "numerical totality" -a very labourious and not a very successful task. Boenninghausen's Pocket Book translated by Dr. T.F., Allen, was the only repertory available - and referring to the materia medica then available did not always help. It was at this time that the great masters and leaders arose, and introduced the system of recognising the "IDENTIFYING SYMPTOMS" from hundreds of "common" symptoms in the materia media. These were to be present in the patient to make the selection a simillimum. Naturally, they had to be "PECULIAR, UNCOMMON and CHARACTERISTIC".

"Great essays on this subject which helped hundreds of beginners and even older people, appeared in the "Hahnnemannian Monthly", the most prestigious of the time. Two were from the pen of Dr. Adolph Lippe "On Characteristic Symptoms" (See Jany, and May 1990 issues of Heritage). Another essay "On Characteristic Symptoms" by Dr. J.H.P. Frost was published just after Dr. Lippe's in "Hah. monthly", in 1874.

"Please note that both the masters did not use the word "Keynotes". Dr. H.N.Guernsey had coined that word in an article in 1868. (See April 1984 issue of Heritage). It was left to Dr. H.C. Allen to join the two words when he published his greatest work: "Keynotes and characteristics".

"Dr. Hering named them "Guiding Symptoms" and created many by the addition of clinical cases which brought out the "verified concomitants" - an extremely valuable branch of the Keynote system".

Now let us see what Drs. Lippe and Frost have to say about the Peculiar and Characteristic symptoms.

What is a Peculiar Symptom? What is it that makes a symptom peculiar? The materia medica is full of

"Common" symptoms, those which are common to many remedies as well as to many diseases. They do not help us a bit. If we remember that in homoeopathy we treat the patient as an individual person, and we do not treat the disease, whatever it may be, it will be clear that we have to look for, hunt for, those symptoms which essentially and definitely pertain to the patient only. In sickness, the symptoms that cannot be explained are often very peculiar-like thirstlessness during high fever, or loquacity during fever; or amelioration of headache from urination; aversion to members of family and loved ones. Asthma better when lying down (Psor.). Painlessness of ulcers (Op.), and so on. Kent makes a significant point which helps us to identify a "Characteristic". He says, "When there are two or three of these peculiar symptoms, they form the CHARACTERISTIC features". He adds, "You cannot individualise unless you have that which characterises". Lippe says: "The truly characteristic symptoms of the patient exist exclusively outside of the pathological groups of symptoms of the discerned disease; nay more, they are symptoms which never necessarily belong to the disease or any form of it, but which appear as absolutely accidental."

We learn the true meaning of a "Characteristic" symptoms more easily and clearly from its application in a case than from a mere description of it. Lippe follows this plan in his article, "The importance of a single symptom" (which must be read as `Single CHARACTERISTIC Symptom'). We summarise his observations:

The importance of a single symptom becomes most apparent when we detect in the patient this single characteristic symptom, corresponding with a similar single characteristic symptom observed by proving a medicine. To illustrate: a case in which an objective symptom indicated the truly specific remedy - a case of very malignant ship fever.

The patient had been sick nine days, lying on his back perfectly unconscious, eyes wide open, glaring, fixed on the ceiling, pupils dilated, cheeks red and hot, mouth wide open, the lower jaw hanging down, tongue and lips dry, black and cracked; picking of bed coverings; pulse 200. Diagnosis: Approaching paralysis of the brain. Should I have administered Morphine, and Opium by the spoonfuls in alternation? The **unconsciousness** could make me think at first of Bell., Hyos., Mur-ac., Op., The **hanging of the lower jaw:** *Ars., Lyc* and *Op.* The **picking of the bed-clothes;** *Ars., Arn, Hyos., Op., and Stram.*

Not being able to select a remedy, I further examined the patient and found that he had passed the *urine involuntarily* all night: had to choose between Arn., Ars., Bell. etc. Upon still further examination, I found on the sheet of the patient, that the urine had made a LARGE DEPOSIT OR RED SAND, resembling BRICK DUST. Here was the OBJECTIVE SYMPTOM CHARACTERISTIC OF THE CASE AND THE REMEDY. *Lyco*. 200th, spoonfuls every two hours in water. Patient then had natural sleep, heavy perspiration - finally recovered fully.

Take the frequently recurring symptoms, "sinking at the epigastrium". This symptom standing alone is of no importance whatever, neither characterising a remedy or any abnormal condition of the system. Lippe examines a number of remedies having this symptom, but with **different variations and modalities,** each modality pointing to a different remedy. This discussion shows how a symptom like "sinking at the epigastrium" can become peculiar in a case and point to different remedies **depending upon the modalities or concomitants.**

Lippe adds : A single symptom is all important if it is the characteristic of the medicine corresponding with the characteristic symptoms of the case to be treated. In as much as we no longer treat diseases... IT IS OUR TASK TO FIND THE SINGLE CHARACTERISTIC SYMPTOM BOTH OF THE PATIENT AND THE REMEDY. If we first arrive at a clear idea of what constitutes the characteristic of medicines, we involuntarily adapt ourselves to easy finding of the characteristic symptoms of the patient..... The **characteristic symptoms of a medicine go through ALL ITS ACTIONS like a red streak.** For instance, all the symptoms which **Aconite** is able to produce are accompanied by "anxiety" and differ in restlessness which is caused by **anguish** under **Ars.**

Some examples of characteristics: Lippe gives more examples:

The "anxiety" of *Acon.* may be termed a general characteristic like the "anguish" of *Ars.*, or the constant aggravation of all the symptoms after sleep under *Lach.* or amelioration in the open, cold air under *Puls;* the amelioration in the cold air alone being equally characteristic to *Iod;* or the aggravation at three a.m. under *Kali-c.*

Besides these *general* characteristics which go through the whole remedy, we observe *special* characteristics, as under Kali-bi. that all the mucous discharges are *stringy,* or under *Phos.* the aggravation of the cough in the cold air.

The single characteristic symptom which becomes all important in a case may comprise the **kind of pains** experienced as under *Apis* (the burning-stinging pains), or the *locality* (as the wrist and ankle under *Ruta*), or the *direction* of the pain from left to right, or from below upwards, or vice versa (*lyc., Lach.*) or *alternating sides* (*Lac.can*), or amelioration from heat (*Ars.*), or amelioration from cold (*Iod.*), or *thirstlessness* under Puls.

The single characteristic symptom becomes all important in well-known diseases, as for instance in whooping cough - in which we must inquire into the character and peculiarities of the cough (but these alone are not sufficient); it is indispensable to inquire about the *time* of the day or night the cough is worse; what are the *concomitant* symptoms, such as vomiting with the cough; the colour and consistency of the *expectoration;* whether the expectoration is copious and threatens suffocation. The single characteristic symptom—most outstanding among those elicited—will enable the prctitioner to select the curative remedy; the name of the disease never will.

Dr. Frost: Let us take a few more points from Dr. Frost. "A case of profuse haemorrhage after abortion at three months. The flow resisted every remedy which was indicated for such a difficulty; Tampon was used as a last resort, but it held for only a few hours. About 3 a.m. the flow returned with redoubled violence. I remembered a similar aggravation had previously occurred at the same time. I immediately gave *NUX VOM.* which otherwise I should never have thought of for haemorrhage. Had no further trouble.

"We must not expect all the characteristic symptoms of a remedy even of the right remedy, to be present in a given case, since different temperaments and constitutions are variously affected in different degrees by the morbific influence; and the resulting symptoms vary in kind, are different in intensity, and in some instances are altogether hindered from appearing.

"Characteristic symptoms, when once well established, may serve to enlarge the sphere of usefulness of the remedies to which they belong - either by encouraging their employment in some cases where the accompanying symptoms were unknown, or *where they have not been recognised hitherto as applicable* to those particular forms of disease. (This reminds me of Dr. Jayesh Shah's case of a very painful goitre, with severe aggravation from any motion (she could not speak at all), cured by *Bryonia* though Bry. is not found in the rubric against "Goitre")

"The most infallible characteristic symptoms are those that appear in groups. And it is believed that whenever a real characteristic symptom of a particular remedy presents itself, however obscurely, *other indications for the same remedy may also be found present* in greater or less abundance. And this is the very function and HIGHEST USE OF THE RECOGNISED CHARACTERISTICS, to lead us to inquire if the remedy they suggest is not the very one most truly indicated by the accompanying symptoms. (We can use this criteria to identify the truly characteristic symptom of the remedies. In other words, the remedy suggested by the truly *characteristic* symptoms will be found to have other characteristic symptoms as well of the patient).

Dr. Frost concludes: "Thus, when an actual GROUP appears of what may be termed the CHARACTERISTIC of a particular remedy, the case is DECIDED AT ONCE; for "in the mouth of two or three witnesses, every word (or thing) shall be established".

We shall cite one more "witness", Dr. E.J.Lee, M.D., about the nature of the Peculiear and Characteristic symptoms. Dr. Lee focusses our attention on Aph. 118, viz. "Every medicine exhibits... specific effects that do not occur from any other medicinal substance in exactly the same way". On a casual examination this seems to give a false impression, for one can hardly recall a single symptom of any drug which is not found in the record of another drug. But on a closer examination of Hahnemann's words we find they are correct. He states that no two drugs produce "specific effects...*in exactly the same way*". For example, the "empty sensation in the abdomen" marked under Phos., or the "bearing down pains"of Sepia, are found with many other remedies; true, but these never occur '*in exactly the same way*'. Thus, the characteristics, that is, the striking, strange, unusual, peculiar' symptoms are the ones which no TWO DRUGS produce 'IN EXACTLY THE SAME WAY'; and these are the symptoms which are to be used in deciding on the simillimum, Therefore, the *characteristic symptoms* of any drug may be termed the *particular effects* of that drug which no other drug produces in a *precisely similar manner.*

Dr. Lee adds: "Hahnemann gives us yet another guide in the study of these characteristics. He tells us that the *mental symptoms* are a surer guide to the proper selection than the pathological. Why are the mental symptoms the most important ones? Because They are the most peculiar, the most striking and uncommon, because they have no pathological or diagnostic value. They are more indicative of the INDIVIDUALITY of the patient than the physical symptoms.

"Totality has to be understood as meaning the TOTALITY OF THE PECULIAR AND UNCOMMON symptoms. They must be covered by the characteristics of a drug. These should be of EQUAL IMPORTANCE in both the drug and the patient.

"Each drug has its particular symptoms which, *taken collectively*, surely indicate that drug. Take Lycopodium, for instance. It has a group of symptoms which, taken together, can always be relied upon to indicate that remedy, though each individual symptom of this group is to be found under other drugs. One could scarcely fail to know what remedy even these few symptoms call for: Aggravation from 4 to 8 p.m.; symptoms going from right to left, especially of the throat; fanlike motion of alae nasi;

PECULIAR, CHARACTERISTIC SYMPTOMS AND KEYNOTES

clear urine depositing a red sandy sediment; backache before urinating; a full, bloated feeling after eating a little; one foot hot, the other cold."

The whole art of prescribing consists in finding for each patient, that drug whose *group of "Specific effects"* are produced by *no other drug* in 'precisely the *similar manner*'.

We have already seen the various differentiating factors—different manner in which symptoms are produced — viz. Mind and disposition; Causation; Concomitants, Conditions of Aggravation or amelioration of the body as a whole (general) and of parts of body (Particulars); location and sensations. These differentiating factors are the particular effects of each drug which no other drug produces in precisely the same manner, in a precise group.

KEYNOTES :- This expressive phrase was coined by Dr. Henry N. Guernnsey in order to simplify the difficult task of identifying the curative remedy in a case even from a few of peculiar symptoms. He found that each medicine presents peculiarities which are different from those of other medicines. These differences by which one remedy is distinguished from another, are the "Keynotes" of the remedy. This description of the distinguishing peculiar symptoms was derived from the analogy of music. The keynote in music is the "the fundamental note or tone around which the whole piece moves." The keynote of one piece of music sets it apart from other pieces even at the first hearing. The keynotes were highly attractive as they did a way with tedious comparisons of drugs (before the detailed Repertories came out) and many brilliant cures were made by means of the keynotes in the hands of Guernsey, Lippe, Allen and others. Guernsey was accused of doing away with "Totality" through this method, but he refuted this by saying that its function is merely suggestive. The keynote is simply the predominating symptoms or feature which directs attention to a remedy which will be found to cover the totality. Knowledge of keynotes narrows down the field of selection, and the prescriber must refer to the repertory or materia medica to verify and complete the comparison.

Kent pointed out that the trouble with keynotes arises when they are misused, and used as sole guides to the remedy. When they are taken as final and the GENERALS do not confirm, then failures will come.

In the preface to his great work on Obstetrics Dr. Guernsey writes about the Keynotes: "It may seem like prescribing for single symptoms, whereas such is not the fact. It is only meant to state some strong characteristic symptom, which will often be found to be the governing symptom, and on referring to the materia medica ALL THE OTHERS WILL BE THERE IF THIS ONE IS. If the most interior or peculiar symptom, or a keynote, is discernible, it will (usually) be found that all the other symptoms of the case will also be found under that remedy which produces this peculiar one". The keynote to a case often consists of a "peculiar combination", as Guernsey put it; strike that *peculiar combination of symptoms*, a characteristic or keynote, and all other features of the case and of the remedy, are easily touched -just as one keynote to the piece of music governs and is in hormony with all the other notes.

Caution in Keynote Prescribing : Dr. F.K. Bellokossy draws attention to the fact that we often hesitate to prescribe a remedy on account of the absence of a certain keynote, which is supposed or regarded as indispensable in every prescription; but which it is not. A keynote of Causticum is its aggravation in dry, clear, fine weather. This is so strongly stressed in text books that we cannot easily free ourself from it. But one day while reading Kent's materia medica he found, "It also has rheumatic complaints aggravated in the warm, damp days, in wet weather, but this is not so striking". From this Bellokossy concludes that while aggr. in dry weather is not an indispensable symptom, it remains precious when present. Arising from this Bellokossy has offered comments on some more keynotes of remedies which are indispensable - i.e.important not only by their presence but also by their absence; viz.

    Anger, impatience and oversensitiveness in Chamomilla
    Scanty menstruation in Graphites
    Warm -bloodedness in Iodine
    Tension for no apparent reason in Nux Vomica.
    Bruised sensation all over the body or its parts in Arnica and in Eupatorium Perfoliatum.
    Weakness, anxiety and restlessness in Arsenic.
    Flabbiness of the tissues in Kali carb.
    Venocity in Carbo veg.
    Pulse not in proportion to temperature in Pyrogen.
    Suppuration in injured parts and oversensitiveness in Hepar.

There are other keynotes, strong, but *dispensable*- important by their presence only, but whose absence has no bearing on the choice of the remedy. e.g.

    Agg. by dryness in Causticum.
    Restlessness in Rhus tox
    Lokquacity in Lachesis
    Sleeps into aggrvation in Lachesis
    Right-sidedness of complaints in Lycopodium
    Thirst for cold drinks in Phosphorus
    Changing of complaints from side to side: Lac can.
    Nausea in Ipecacuanha
    Music causes weeping in Graph.
    Complaints go upward: Led.

8 | Perceive the MOST uncommon (unusual), peculiar symptom

H.C. Allen's two cases will throw further light on how, when confronted with a number of peculiar symptoms, we have to select the MOST striking and uncommon, even rare, symptom as the deciding factor in the choice of the remedy. He writes:

> **A case** report by Dr. Farrington (N.Y.State transactions) illustrates this point in which there were many "characteristic" symptoms, and the difficulty was to decide upon the one most peculiar and uncommon. "Palpitation of heart worse lying down at night. Frontal headache. Sensation of a load in stomach after even a light meal unless she chews some soft substances. No inclination for the bowels to move; is compelled to take Cascara Sagrada; has "lived on purgatives for years". Faints in a warm room; always better in the open air, even though she is chilly. Cries easily; constantly depressed. Cannot urinate without getting down on "all fours". Urine deposits a red sandy sediment".

Here are characteristics of *Bry.*, *Lyc.*, *Nux-v.*, *Puls.*, but the most uncommon symptom is the position the patient is compelled to assume in order to urinate, and which is found under *Pareira brava*, and under no other drug. Its use was followed by the most satisfactory result.

Another case: A lady suffering from severe congestive headache. The attack was attributed to some mental excitement to which she had been subjected in the afternoon. The pain began in the evening and thinking to obtain relief, she retired early. The Violence of the attack soon compelled her to leave the bed and walk the floor to obtain relief. The pain was pressing, throbbing, bursting, as if the head was too full. The head, face and neck were red and hot; the carotids throbbed violently. Felt "Would become insane if it continued another hour". The only relief she could obtain was by pressing the sides of her head with both hands and walking as rapidly as possible from end to end of the suite of three rooms. The congestion, etc. certainly pointed to **Bell.** but the manner of obtaining relief from rapid motion - the most uncommon symptom - promptly excluded **Bell.** Any remedy that would cure her **must contain among its totality, this peculiar symptom** which is a characteristic of *Sepia*. A few pellets of *Sep.200* in sponfuls of water every ten minutes relieved her before the third dose arrived. She fell asleep and next day she was as well as usual.

9. Take POSITIVE symptoms irrespective of the "drug picture"

We often come across cases which do not present the typical "text-book drug picture" of a remedy, but demand that remedy by sheer number of geniune indications, worked out by Repertory or Materia Medica. What shall we do? Margaret Tyler throws light on this problem and show the way. She says:

> "Typical cases are child's play; the elderly woman, a hearty eater who likes fat and is famished at 10-11 a.m. , who feels the heat and sticks her burning soles out of bed at night, shreiks for *Sulphur,* and you must indeed be deaf to miss her cry. She will respond every time, whatever ails her, and will return once or twice a year for any little ailment or flagging health, just to get the fresh stimulus which keeps her going happily. Or,

> "The tall slender, sensitive child, to whom darkness and thunder are terrors; who prefers highly seasoned foods and salt to the sickly sweets that appeal to her fellows, and whose eyes gleam at the mere mention of ices; here, it is very hard to miss her magic - *Phosphorus.*

"But there are plenty of **atypical** people; a *Pulsatilla* who likes fat; a desperate acute *Arsenicum* even that is neither restless nor anxious - one comes across such cases once in a way. Quite a number of patients fails to conform to any remedy in common use and within our easy ken, presenting the typical symptoms at our finger-ends. It is important to remember in these cases what Dr. Clarke insisted on:

> "IT IS THE POSITIVE SYMPTOMS that decide the remedy. Negative symptoms are of no use, i.e., the fact that a person has a certain symptom, is all important and the fact that he has no symptoms that **you think he ought to have,** if a certain remedy is to fit him, is QUITE UNIMPORTANT".

"Any person may require any remedy in his acute sickness. and it is useless to say: "He cannot need this or that because "he has not put up what one (rightly) considers the characteristic symptoms of a drug. But always, it is the POSITIVE symptoms of the patient at the moment that demand a certain remedy, and the negative symptoms must not be allowed to call us off.

"A doctor, himself a pretty experienced prescriber, was suffering from a virulent cold, first affecting nose and frontal sinuses, then a sharp attack of laryngitis. His symptoms were (i) Burning pains (with such septic colds); (ii) Sputum sticky; (iii) Sputum bloody; (iv) Sweat at night; (v) worse uncovering. These symptoms, characteristic of his acute sickness suggested Phos; and after a few doses of Phos.30 they all disappeared, and he was suddenly well.

"But he had no 'Phos. symptoms'. He liked being alone, had no fear of the dark, no craving for salt—did not eat it even with eggs—had no thirst, no desire for cold drinks — though he did like ices when set before him. These were NEGATIVE — could not contra-indicate by their absence".

"The typical drug is magic; but the quite ATYPICAL drug, when called for in sickness by unusual POSITIVE symptoms, and even when "contra-indicated" (as it seems) by the general symptoms of the patient, is the one which when given will give the desired result - in the usual sudden brilliant and unmistakeable way".

10   Totality of symptoms

It is time that we examine what we really mean by Totality. Let us turn to Stuart Close for a clear and succint elucidation. Hahnemann says (Org. Aph.6): "The ensemble or totality of these available signs or symptoms, represents in its full extent the disease itself; that is, they constitute the true and only form, which the mind is capable of conceiving". Totality represents the disease; as also the remedy, as language represents thought.

1) Totality means, first, the totality of each individual symptom. Every complete symptom has three essential elements: location, sensation and modality. A single symptom is a fact with its history, its origin, its progress or direction and its conditions.

2) Totality means all the symptoms of the case which are capable of being logically combined into a harmonious and consistent whole, having form, coherency and individuality. It is more (and may be less) than the mere numerical totality; it includes "concomitants" or the form in which the symptoms are grouped. Hahnemann calls totality (Aph.7) the image (or picture) reflecting outwardly the internal essence of the disease, i.e., of the suffering life force." It must express an idea.

3) The totality is not a numerical aggregate, in the same way as the idea or thought cannot be a numerical aggregate of a jumble of words. Only when the words are joined coherently can they

TOTALITY OF SYMPTOMS 45

present an idea or thought. In short, *the totality must represent the picrure the disease as well as of the drug.* The characteristic symptoms when brought together must form an organic whole as an individuality, an identity which may be seen and recognised as we recognise the personality of a friend.

4) The same idea underlies the phrase, "Genius of the Remedy". in the sense of being the dominant influence, or the essnetial principle of the remedy, which gives it its individuality. The materia medica thus becomes portrait gallery of diseases, a "Rogues" Gallery by means of which we may identify the thieves who steal our health and comfort, and bring them to justice.

11 The Contribution of Dr. J.T. Kent to the advancement of Homoeopathy

The advent of Kent as a leading thinker, teacher and practitioner of Homoeopathy led to a great resurgence in the practice of homoeopathy on the lines laid down by Hahnemann. Dr. Richard Hughes dominated Homoeopathy in England for fifty years, but after his death when Dr. Margaret Tyler and Sir John Wier returned to England after studyinng under Kent in the U.S.A., it did not take long for Kent's teachings to strike roots and spread in England, and from there to other parts of the world. Hughes adopted certain principles of Homoeopathy, e.g. the law of similars, in his teachings and practice, but was dead set against any potency higher than the 6th. He believed in pathological prescribing, and put in enormous labour to compile his "Cyclopaedia of Drug Pathogenecy" by what he called "purifying" the Materia Medica Pura. His aim was to make homoeopathy easy and acceptable to Allopaths. Thus his book came to be called the "homoeopathic milk for allopathic babies." The teachings of Kent completely reversed this scene, and also considerably modified Boenninghausen's evaluation of symptoms in the search for the simillimum. He went back to the teachings of the Organon, and thanks to his able elucidation of the various Aphorisms in the Organon, (vide his Lectures on Homoeopathic Philosophy), his brilliant Lectures on Materia Medica, revealing his keen insight into the drug pictures, together with his clinical achievements,

THE CONTRIBUTION OF Dr. J.T. KENT

Hahnemannian homoeopathy is today occupying a commanding height. His Repertory of the materia medica has made it easy for practitioners to easily find the simillimum, subject only to their correct grasp of the philosophy and acquiring the skill for putting it into practice. All his writings, such as "Use of the Repertory", and "Kent's Minor Writings", besides the three books mentioned earlier must be studied again and again if one wishes to be a master prescriber as Kent was. We shall give the highlights from his teachings in brief, including his departure from Boenninghausen's method.

Kent classified the symptoms in three classes: Generals, Particulars and Common. The Generals relate to the whole person, in narrating which the patient uses the word "I"; - e.g. "I am depressed", "I have no appetite"; "I pass sleepless nights", and so on. The Generals are divided into two parts. Mental symptoms are the highest ranking generals if clear and outstanding, as they represent the person in his entirety. Next are the Physical Generals: reaction of the patient as a whole to heat and cold, cravings and aversions to items of food and drink. Modalities of aggravation or amelioration in relation to the whole body, such as before, or during, or after sleep, stool, eating, menses; periodicity of complaints and the time of aggravation of complaints; position in sleep, etc., etc. A list of Physical Generals is given in Appendix 'A'

The common symptoms are those which are large in number and are common to many diseases and to many remedies. It is difficult to individualise with their help, unless they are modified (qualified) by Modalities of aggravation or amelioration or other circumstances, or by concomitants or other peculiar symptoms.

Some pointed observations of Kent are given hereunder:

Only when the vital principle is disturbed can it give

to the organism its abnormal sensations and incline it to the irregular actions we call disease.

Morbid disturbances can be perceived solely by means of the expression of disease in the disturbed sensations and functions...... if these were not present, we would have no means of putting the patient in freedom.

To think of remedies for cancer is confusion - but to think of remedies for the PATIENT who appears to have cancer is orderly, and you will be astonished to know what wonderful changes will take place in these conditions when remedies that correspond to the conditions before the cancer began are administered.

When the strong symptoms are all gathered together, the physician in studying the case must separate out those things that were observed years ago from those things that are observed today, noting how they have changed and why changed. He must learn the changes all along the line, from beginning to end.

The real study of sick man is the meditation on his symptoms, and to become wise in symptoms is to become an able prescriber.

Causes are continued into effects (i.e. causes continue in ultimates); all ultimates to a great extent contain the cause or the beginnnings. When symptoms manifest themselves into a disease of the ovary, removal of that ovary does not remove the cause; it will manifest itself through some other part of the body, perhaps the other ovary. It is a serious matter to remove any organ through which the disease is manifested. A tuberculous condition of the lungs may remain in a very quiet state so long as a fistula in ano keeps on discharging, but once that vent is closed, immediately there is a cropping out of the disease by infiltration of the lungs, and the patient comes to an early death.

Cure of disease means permanent removal of the totality of the symptoms, thus removing the cause and turning DISORDER into ORDER, and as a consequence the **results** of disease are removed. The expert prescriber has fixed in his mind the image of the sick man before he takes up a book or thinks or a remedy. He masters the sickness before he asks himself what is its likeness.

Some more POINTERS FROM KENT:

1) The Keynotes are often characteristic symptoms, but if the keynotes are taken as final, and GENERALS DO NOT CONFIRM, then will come the failures.

    If you see the keynotes of Arsenicum, next see to it that the patient is chilly, sensitive to air, fearful, restless, weak, pale, must have the picture on the wall hung straight, and ARS will cure.

2) Nothing can take the place of mastering the materia medica. My lectures on Materia Medica give the plan of study for each remedy. The "Guiding Symptoms" (of Hering) give the plan of study for characteristics and grades as a referende book.

    The "Encyclopaedia" (of T.F. Allen) is the book of reference for a full study of provings. The doctor that does any of these will never grow into an artist. I am an enemy of all short-cuts to science and art. Prolonged and deep effort, drudgery, only can make an artist in healing or music.

3) There is need to develop the genius of men and women in the art of healing. Some try to shorten the work by the use of keynotes, but that system is destruction to the art, and it is the cultivation of memory instead of the UNDERSTANDING.

    It is not the man who remembers much that makes the artist, but the one who KNOWS and UNDERSTANDS. The artist knows how to meet every emergency, but the memoriser has forgotten what he has memorised and NEVER UNDERSTOOD.

4) Try to make use of the method of working out such cases as are obscure by the only individualising method known to us, viz. the repertory, for each patient.

5) If you find certain PECULIAR symptoms running through every region of the body, they will become GENERALS as well as particulars. Things that modify all parts of the organism are those that relate to the general state. Anything that the individual predicates of himself is also a general.

6) When a man says, "I was wakeful last night," he is predicating something of himself, and hence it is a general. You might say that the mind merely dreamed, but the MIND IS THE MAN. We see how important sleep and dreams become in the anemnesis of a case. The same principle applies to the MENSTRUAL function of a woman. The special senses are also closely related to the whole man; smells that are grateful or disagreeable become generals.

7) The things that relate to the man are the ones to be SINGLED out in the anemnesis and marked first. Sometimes when you have figured out the anemnesis of the GENERALS, you will possibly settle upon three remedies, or possibly upon one.

8) In ninety - nine cases out of a hundred you can LEAVE OUT THE PARTICULARS, for the particulars are usually contained within the generls. If there is but one remedy that has the numerous generals, and covers those generals absolutely and clearly and strongly, that will be the remedy that will cure the case. NOTHING IN PARTICULARS CAN CONTRADICT GENERALS, but ONE STRONG GENERAL CAN OVER-

RULE ALL THE PARTICULARS you can gather up. "Aggravation from heat" will throw out *Arsenicum* from consideration in any case.

9) A woman complains of prolapsus. This is a common symptom with a dozen remedies. How will you pick out of that group of remedies, the one that will cure this lady? You must then study the GENERALS AND THE PARTICULARS of the patient, the generals always FIRST. If it is a *Nux vomica* patient with prolapsus of the uterus, what will make you see *Nux* in it? She would be chilly; full of coryza, with stuffing up of the nose in a warm room; she would be very irritable, snappish, wants to kill somebody, to throw her child into the fire, to kill her husband; may be she is constipated, with ineffectual urging to stool. You at once see that she has the generals of *Nux.*, and whatever particulars SHE HAS ARE IN HARMONY WITH THOSE GENERALS. So you *go from generals to particulars*.

10) Unless the symptoms that CHARACTERISE the patient are brought on record (through careful observation and interrogation), the physician should not be surprised at failure. The remedy must be similar to the symptoms of the patient as well as the pathognomonic symptoms of his disease in order to cure.

12   Kent's Repertory-How to use it

As stated earlier, Boenninghausen did not differentiate between modalities and sensations pertaining to parts of body (Particulars) and those pertaining to the individual as a whole. Kent was of the opinion that the modalities pertaining to the parts cannot and should not be applied to the person and raised to the rank of generals. Yet he said, "Our generals were well worked out by Boenninghausen and much overdone, as he generalised many rubrics that were purely particulars, the use of which as generals is misleading and ends in failure. The success coming from Boenninghausen's Pocket Book is due to the arrangement whereby generals can be quickly made use of to furnish madalities for individual symptoms, whether general or particular. This feature is preserved in my repertory, as all know who use it.

"The new Repertory is produced to show forth all the particulars, each symptoms with the circumstances connected with it. It is in its infancy....The author is devoting his life to the growth and infilling and perfecting of this work...and begs all true workers" for help in this work. What do these remarks show? They show that although Kent gave top rank to Mentals, with the Physical Generals coming next, he gave equal importance to particulars provided they are qualified by modalities. Kent's repertory gives a huge number of verified by modalities. Kent's repertory gives a huge number of verified, qualified Particulars but they are yet "scanty" (that is incomplete) according to Kent. But where we are able to locate one, the results have been truly marvellous, subject only to the condition that they do not "contradict the Generals". This much, in brief, is about the construction of the repertory. Kent's advice as to how to use his Repertory may be briefly sumed up as follows:

The first and highest thought in homoeopathy is the individual. Our work is individualisation.

I once planned a short-cut with Cards, but I soon saw that I must work out every case, every patient, on his own merit in each and every case, making use of the fullest repertory accessible, curtailing nothing lest I miss something important.

I prescribed for twenty-five to forty patients in one and half hours and never neglected anybody. This can be done by anybody unless he works uphill with his cases.

A doctor should know GENERALS, COMMON SYMPTOMS and PARTICULARS to the fullest if he wants to save work, so that he can use them quickly if he has a large business.

When looking over a list of symptoms, first of all discover 3,4,5,or 6 symptoms that are "strange, rare and peculiar". *Work these out first.* These are the HIGHEST GENERALS, as they apply to the patient himself. Then find out which one of this list is most like the rest of the symptoms, common and particular. To individualise between these few remedies you must have the fullest repertory that can be found. The symptoms you settle upon must be such that CANNOT BE OMITTED in each individual.

Do not expect a remedy that has the generals must have all the little symptoms. It is a waste of time to run out all the little symptoms. Learn to omit the useless, common particulars.

Get the strong, strange, peculiar symptoms, and then SEE TO IT THAT THERE ARE NO GENERALS IN THE CASE THAT OPPOSE OR CONTRADICT.

Those wishing to have more details are referred to Glen Bidwell's "How to use the Repertory" and Margaret Tyler's "Repertorising". A few excerpts from Tyler's "Repertorising" would be in order.

1. A lot of time and labour in repertorising can be saved if one follows the GRADING of symptoms. Mental symptoms are of first grade. *A strongly marked* mental symptom will always rule out any number of poorly marked symptoms of LESSER GRADE. One should combine two rubrics that practically amount ot the same thing; e.g. *aversion to company* and *better alone*, though different, are sometimes difficult to sort out. Similarly "worse in the darkness" and "fear of darkness".

2. Next come the Physical Generals (Time, Modalities, etc.) but they have got to be in CAPITALS (bold letters) or in italics in the PATIENT AS WELL AS IN THE REPERTORY, to take this rank; or to be safely used as eliminating symptoms. This means that the first One or Two symptoms which are to be used as *"Eliminating Symptoms"* (to `eliminate' or throw out those remedies in the *remaining* rubrics, which are not found in the *first two* rubrics, MUST BE in bold type or italics. The first two "eliminating rubrics" naturally have to be INDISPENSABLE, strong, well-marked and characteristic, to the case. If less important rubrics are used as "eliminative". the curative remedy itself may be thrown out.

3. The third grade General symptoms are Cravings and Aversions, not mere dislikes, but *longings* and likings; in *corresponding types* in the patient and the rubrics.

For instance, if your patient is only a little restless, *Ars.* and *Rhus tox,* superlatively restless remedies, will be rather contra-indicated.

4. Go for the patient as a live entity, revealed by his general and mental symptoms in chief. The whole is greater than its part. But, in their position of secondary importance, you must go into the Particulars all the same, if only to confirm your choice of the drug. Among the particulars, your first-grade symptoms will be those which are peculiar, *unusual unexpected, or unaccountable.*

5. If you are to be a good prescriber, study the drugs in the same way as you know people with their whims, fancies, cheerful or sad, loquacious or taciturn, who crave sweets or salt or meat or hate them; quarrelsome and fault finding or affectionate and mild, etc.

6. If you have a patient who is predominantly WORSE FROM HEAT, here is an Eliminating Symptom for you. Ruthlessly cut out all the remedies that are chilly. None of them you need write down at all. And so on, down all the remaining rubrics, mental, general and particular, you will carry that great eliminating symptom. For instance, with just two important symptoms alone (worse from heat and worse from consolation), which have got to be in *equal type in the patient and in the drug,* you have reduced your area of search to *Lil-tig., Nat-mur* and *Plat....* If you get such marked eliminating symptoms to begin with, see what a comparatively small number of drugs you have to carry down through all the rubrics, and how much easier and quicker it is to get your remedy.... you will find that one drug stands out more and more pre-eminently-it maynot be in all the rubrics, *but it has got to be in all the important ones,* those best marked in the patient, and of highest grade in the repertory.

7. Totality means the CHARACTERISTIC TOTALITY; cease counting fingers and toes. A drug picture to be complete, does not consist of strings of little symptoms, but of BROAD OUTLINES OF MENTAL AND PECULIAR symptoms-peculiar to one drug and distinguishing it from all others. Get the strong, strange, peculiar symptoms, and then SEE TO IT THAT THERE ARE NO GENERALS IN THE CASE THAT OPPOSE OR CONTRADICT.

8. Many drugs can be got only by reading and studying their GENIUS. One of the veterans used to lay down his own law: "Read a drug a day, and two on Sundays."

9. When in a case there is a **strongly marked** mental symptom, use **that as an Eliminating Symptom** and while going through the remaining rubrics, record only those that have this mental symptom.

10. The amount of time and labour involved in finding the remedy be means of the REPERTORY may be immensely lightened if we realise the Grading of Symptoms - their relative value — and by using the highest grades as **"Eliminating Symptoms."**

13   WHAT TO DO WHEN STRONG MENTALS ARE NOT AVAILABLE?

It is all very well to say, "Start with the Mentals and end with the Particulars". Unfortunately, in quite a number of cases we are not able to observe or elicit any marked, outstanding mentals on which to base a prescription. What do we do then? The masters who laid down the "Ideal method" referred to were not unaware of this difficulty. Even Kent who was second to none in his emphasis of Mentals, as the highest general which should ever guide us, illustrated a solution of this problem in his article, "Use of the Repertory". He presents a problem where the Particulars in the Repertory do not contain the qualifying modalities. He takes the case of "Writer's cramp." He says, "If we should take" Writer's cramp" and say no more about it, you would have only a limited number of remedies to look to for cure. But our **resources are unlimited.** When examined into, it means cramps in fingers, hand or arms, or all three. Sometimes numbness and tingling of one or all three; sometimes sensation of paralysis in one or all three. In all of these conditions from writing or worse while writing. these scanty rubrics may or may not show the remedy. We may then proceed as follows: Use the General groups of remedies (at the **head** of the rubrics) Cramp in the fingers, hand and wrist, or such parts as are affected. Similarly use the **General group** against numbness of fingers; and the **General group** against Sensation of paralysis. Now turn to the **General rubric** against "exertion"' in "Generalities" as writing is nothing but prolonged exertion. Compare all these, and you will be able to find the remedy for the complaint. It is using a **general rubric** in a proper manner. (It will be seen that this process is not different from that laid down by Boenninghausen).

Dr. W.A.Yingling, a strong advocate of the use of mental symptoms, offers his solution to a similar problem: "Unfortunately in many cases the "more prominent, peculiar symptoms" are not to be found, no matter how carefully one searches for them. When this is the fact - and I find it in a large proportion of the cases - I have to resort to other means. I am speaking particularly of chronic cases in which the symptoms are seldom clear cut and striking. Under these circumstances, I have found many times that what has been called the "completed symptom" gives very satisfactory results. I mean by this that after taking careful notes of the case and **arranging the symptoms in the order in which they appeared,** I then select those **"which were the latest to appear, for to those especially should the remedy be similar".** These latest symptoms can usually be arranged under the following heads: (1) Location, the part affected; (ii) how affected; pain, swelling, (sensations) (iii) Modalities. Work out the remedies for these rubrics by the process of elimination, to arrive at 3 or 4 remedies. Often the concomitants are also included. Turn to the materia medica to determine which one of them this case requires".

A few cases from my practice will show how Kent's Repertory can be used, (without necessarily going into the mental symptoms), by taking the most prominent, but peculiar symptoms.

CASE 1 : A lady, 37, came with a complaint of scaly dandruff. While taking the case she disclosed that her real anxiety was about bleeding from the right nipple during menses. She was advised operaiton of the papilloma. She had severe mastitis after her first child-birth 10 years ago, and since then had been having pain in the breast during every menstruation. On the basis of "Inflammation, mammae" (KR.836). Tumour mammae (882), Cancer mammae suspected (824), Pain, mammae during menses (846) and Skin, eruptions, Scaly (1318), she was given *Phytolacca* 200, with relief of all her complaints within a month. Phyt. is not found against "Bleeding nipples" (824) and "Dandruff" (114).

CASE 2 : A young man of 28 complained that during coition, just at the time when semen is about to be ejected the volumptuous sensation is suddenly arrested, the semen is not emitted and the penis becomes relaxed. He felt miserable for the next two days and became indifferent to everything. I could not find a corresponding rubric in the Repertory. Fortunately, while studyinng *Magnetic polus australis* for a case of "ingrowing toe nail", for which it is well-known, I came across the exact condition of this case in Allen's Keynotes. This remedy completely relieved the young man of this embarrassing complaint.

CASE 3 : A lady of 37 used to have severe menorrhagia every month, so much that she was afraid she will die. Even allopathic injections proved unavailing. She was worse when lying down and instantly relieved when sitting up. Based on the rubric "Menses, copious, agg. lying (only on this rubric) she was given *Kreosotum* 200 with almost instant relief. Later on the husband revealed that the couple used to experience sensation of burning during coition, as graphically described in Kent's Lectures on Materia Medica.

CASE 4 : A lady doctor about 30 came from N.India with a history of 3 abortions, every time at the end of the fourth month. This time only 15 days were left for 4 months. As a case of "incompetent Os" she had undergone the Shirodkar Stitch, but still she felt a certain movement in the uterus and uncertainty as if she is going to abort again. Apis 200, followed by 10M-single dose-after 36 hours saved her from the calamity. Indications :Page 241 of Dr.W.A.Yingling's Accoucher's Emergency Manual. Allen's Keynotes gives under Apis "Diarrhoea involuntary, as though anus was wide open (Phos); also K.R.623 "Rectum open: sensation and P.633 Rectum relaxed. I thought to myself, if Apis has wide open rectum (incompetent), it can also have, by analogy, Os an organ contiguous to rectum wide open (incompetent). Apis 10M was the perfect simillimum. I have seen this effect in two more cases subsequently. (Rember : Apis 10M for Incompetent Os).

CASE 5 . A lady, 60, was in hospital for hydronephrosis. She developed retention of urine, and had to be given catheter once. She could not pass urine in the bed pan, she could do it only if she stood bent forward, but she was too weak to be taken to the toilet. *Chimaphilla Umbellata* 200 put and end to this trouble. Indications: "Urination retarded,can only pass urine while standing with feet wide apart and body inclined forward" (K.R.661); and Boericke's Materia Medica page 193.

CASE 6 : A young man aged 32 complained of cramping pain in the abdomen, especially hypogastrium, every night between 2 and 4 a.m. for the last six months, relieved only by bending forward. The pain came on gradually and also subsided gradually. He did not have the pain at any other time even in day time. Indications : KR.1377 and p.512 "Pain appears gradually and disappears gradually. Pain cramping in abdomen better from pressure (KR.559).

WHAT TO DO WHEN STRONG MENTALS ARE NOT AVAILABLE?   61

Cramping pain in hypogastrium (KR.576). Periodicity (KR.1390) - the pain rubrics did not give specific time of aggravation. *Stannum* 200 a few doses relieved.

CASE 7 : A lady complained that her 12 years old dog was not able to walk because of weakness of its hind legs. They could not take it out for the morning walk. Rubric : (KR.1228) Lower extremities, weakness, paralytic: *Cocculus* in the highest grade. *Cocculus* 200 cured the dog with just three or four doses.

CASE 8 : A young man around 40 complained of vertigo, high blood pressure and extreme exhaustion. He had found that he has this extreme weakness every time following coition. Indications: Weakness, coition after (KR.1416). To select one remedy out of the several in this rubric he was asked about his history of past illnesses and general modalities. he had suffered from typhoid for a month several years ago, and since then had found the hot weather, especially summer unbearable. On this basis *Selenium* was selected and a few doses were given in 200th potency. He felt better almost immediately and his vertigo as well as Blood Pressure came down in the next few days.

CASE 9: A 40 years old lady with pain in the left thumb joint, which prevented her from using that thumb. No history of sprain, yet the pain partook of the nature of a "sprain". Various remedies like Rhus tox, Ruta, Arnica, failed to help; not even the help of an orthopaedic doctor. At last *Strontium Carb* 10M cured in three doses, one daily. Ref. Phatak's Materia Medica: "Rheumatic pains. Chronic sprains" (p.563). also Boericke's Mat. Medica.

14   Why are Particulars less important in remedy selection?

Then we come to the particulars, the things for which the patient comes for treatment, say a hip-joint case. Kent says: Most of my cases were cured by remedies NOT IN THE HIP-JOINT LIST. This list contains those remedies that have been observed to cure hip-joint cases, but this remedy with which I cure a patient who has hip-joint trouble may not cure another hip-joint case. Hence it is not in the list, nor is it included as a clinical symptom.

"A man with a rectal ulcer was advised to be operated on to relieve copious haemorrhages from the rectum. He came to me before deciding on the operation. His persistent mental symptom was the need to exercise intense restraint to prevent himself from destroyinng his own life. *Natrum sulph.* has this symptom, but it has no rectal ulcer recorded. A few other symptoms present, together with the strong mental symptom, led to the use of *Nat. Sulph.* and he had no more haemorrhages.

By beginning the investigation in relation to the patient, you may find none of the particulars in the remedy selected, but the remedy cures the patient, and the particulars disappear."

Why is this so? Has not Hahnemann said that every organism is a unity. It is **indivisible**. The parts do not suffer alone, and the whole organism is in a disease state.

WHY ARE PARTICULARS LESS IMPORTANT IN REMEDY SELECTION?

Therefore, it should be possible to understand the condition of the whole organism by understanding any of its parts. Conversely, we do not treat a local malady as a separate entity but as a part of the whole. In fact, Pierre Schmidt has described the relation existing between parts of the body and the whole organism as follows:

> The parts and the whole share the same vicissitudes and pursue the same destiny. So one can understand that from the minute detail of the system, a well-informed and wise observer is enabled to gather the whole just as the naturalist recreates the unknown beast on the mere examination of the skull or a teeth...To those with the eyes to see, each organ reveals the entire organism. Each point of the economy should be studied in its relationship to the whole, and could thus furnish precious data.

Does this mean that Kent was wrong in giving the last place to, if not even ignoring, the particulars? Really speaking though what Pierre Schmidt said was theoretically true it is not the whole truth. The fact is that one will go wrong if he starts analysing a case for repertorisation or finding the remedy by taking the particulars first because of a number of reasons. Firstly, during the provings the remedies were not pushed to the point where they could develop particular or pathological symptoms. Secondly, the Particular symptoms are mostly found to have been the individual reaction of the provers concerned, without any certainty that they are pure symptoms universally present in all or most of the provers. Thirdly, the Particular (local symptoms) are common to many remedies and many patients with the result that they cannot help us at all to differentiate one remedy from another. Yet Kent did not ignore Particulars provided they were qualified by modalities of aggravation or amelioration or by concomitannts or by extension from one part to another. "There are strange and rare symptoms even in parts of the body" he says. Then again he says, clinically verified "remedies may be added to the scanty list of particulars.... and in this manner our Repertory will grow into usefullness. This is the legitimate use of clinical symptoms... to the end that our scanty particulars may be built up". All this only means that the Particulars being "scanty" cannot be given the highest rank, but if they are supported by modalities, etc. with repeated clinical confirmation (three marks in the repertory), they should not be ignored.

On the other hand, it has been repeatedly found from experience that a remedy which has the outstanding mentals and physical generals can be relied upon to constitute the simillimum, even without taking into account the particulars.

15 State of disposition and mind chiefly determines selection

We have so far studied the relative value of the various class of symptoms, viz. modalities, location and sensations, causation and concomitants emphasised by Boenninghausen and Boger; then the General, Particulars and Peculiar symptoms of Kent, who regarded outstandinng mental symptoms as the highest ranking Generals. We shall now carry Kent's emphasis on the paramount importance of mental symptoms one or two steps forward. We shall see how we can understand the state of mind and disposition, deriving our inspiration from Hahnemann's Aphorisms in the "Organon" as well as the observations of Dr. Rajan Sankaran born of his keen insight and deep thinking over his clinical experiences.

In Aphorism 211 Hahnemann clearly affirms that "the state of disposition of the patient often chiefly determines the selection of the homoeopathic remedy, as being decidedly a characteristic symptom which can least of all remain concealed from the accurately observing physician". He reiterates this point in the next Aph. 212 and adds, "there is no powerful medicinal substance... which does not very notably alter the state of the disposition and mind... and every medicine does so *in a different manner*". In Aphorisms 118 and 119 we find Hahnemann asserting that "each of these substances produces alterations in the health of human beings in a peculiar, different, determinate manner, so as to preclude the possibility of confounding one with another". If, therefore, the disposition and mind of each remedy is different from other remedies, how do we find so many remedies against most of the rubrics in the repertory, and how can we differntiate them on the basis of mentals themselves? One answer to this problem is that the symptoms of mind of any remedy do not come under one rubric alone, but come under a group of two, three or more rubrics and if we compare remedies in the form of a chart under these several rubrics of mind, we shall find that the components of mind symptoms of different remedies are not the same, and they do differ, with one or more important symptoms being present or absent. In short the nature of the components (group) decides in favour of one remedy against another. If, for example, we want to differentiate between *Cham.* and *Cina,* we will find that some rubrics contain both of them, while some have only one and not the other; but for the comparison to be accurate, we need to have taken the case in full, and if we miss one important symptom we may go wrong. This is the trouble when we base our selection of the remedy on "symptoms" alone. That is why Kent said: "It is not the man who remembers much that makes the artist, but the one who knows and understands the materia medica. The artist knows how to meet every emergency, but the memoriser has forgotten what he has memorised and never understood. The artistic method thus leans heavily on an *understanding of the drug picture*- the esence, the core or the grand characteristics of the drugs.

How do we understannd the remedy, its core? This is obviously done through understanding the "altered state of the mind and disposition" since the state of mind alone truly represents the man himself. Chamber's 20th Century Dictionary defined "state" as "position, condition, situation, circumstances at any time"; and it defines "disposition" as the "natural tendency or temper". It is not possible to understannd the natural tendency or condition, situation or circumstance of a patient, by asking a few questions about his anger or mildness, shock or grief, inter-personal relations with members of family or at work, etc. We have to acquire a thorough understanding of the patient's psyche (temper, condition or situation), and can do so only by going deep into his life situation and, while doing so, not merely observing the symptoms he indirectly expresses, but by empathising with him and grasping the basic import of the entire situation in which he is placed, especially his emotional disturbances as expressed through Anxiety, disappointment, fright, forsaken or neglected feeling injustice, insult etc. etc.

Understanding the mental set-up of a person is like understanding the thought or the idea presented in a paragraph. A paragraph represents the full description of a thought. Neither the words which make up the sentences, nor the sentences separately can represent the full idea or thought, though the words and sentences are important by themselves. The symptoms are like the words and sentences. How do we get the key idea of a paragraph? This we do by understanding the few key expressions of the dominant ideas in it after concentrating and poring over the entire paragraph. We go through this same process for identifying the state of Mind and Disposition. In short, to understand the dominent thought, the state of Mind and Disposition, we have to look behind the "face totality" or the "surface symptoms".

Experience through taking the case and trying to understand the mind and disposition of patients teaches that the "State of Mind" is more often a "submerged state", submerged deep in the psyche. To bring this submerged state to the conscious level we have to ask the patient to dig into his/her past from childhood and bring to the surface the various incidents in his life which have shaped his emotions, feelings, his attitude to life, to persons and to situations - all of which have made him what he is feels and does today. In case he cannot do this to our satisfaction, we shall have to glean his basic features through the "straws in the wind", some rare and unwittingly uttered flashes or incidents which he narrates while stating his case. We must be ever alert to seize upon such flashes. When the patient describes his hopes and disappointments, his feelings, griefs, anxieties, fears, etc. we have to perceive the *emotional red thread* running through all his narration. That red thread will represent his "state of mind and disposition". We shall illustrate this process through a few cases.

CASE 1: A 17 years old girl was brought by her parents with the complaint of having strange hallucinations - that she is pregnant, that the housing society's watchmen are threatening to rape her, that her father is in legue with the police to keep a watch on her, etc. She did not have her menses since three months; was suspicious of everyone and did not talk to anyone except her father, etc. She was gives Hyos., Stram and Lach., each time on the basis of her complaints/symptoms. Except for restoration of menses after Lachesis there was no change in her hallucinations. In view of this, her past life was gone into from childhood to ascertain her natural disposition of mind as well as the altered state of mind. The lateste *cause* of her complaint was believed to be failure in B.com examination. She was **adamant** in preparing for B.Com as well as Cost & Works Accounts examination and as she was working hard for them against her parents' advice, she felt chagrined when she failed and did not tell her parents about her failure, and instead started behavinng funnily. From her childhood she had nursed the **ambition** of attaining high qualifications, and compared herself to her father and uncles who were all Engineerrs well placed in life. We concluded that this failure came as a big **disappointment** to her. Even during her current mental troubles, she was saying that she wants to **learn Karate.** This situation was converted to rubrics : Ardent (she put in very hard work to fulfill her ambition) SR.101; Ambition: SR 24; A.F. disappointment : SR. 17; A.F.Ambition, deceived : SR. 13. *Nux vomica* revealed by this ardent disposition and disappointed mental state, given in 10M three doses completely cured her. Remedies given on the basis of symptoms of delusions had failed totally.

CASE 2: A young man of 30 complained of peeling of skin with cracks in winter. Also sever he migraine since 12 years. The throbbing headache was worse before examination, mental exertion, heat of sun. It was accompanied by intense photophobia, and amelioration by sleep in a dark room. He had to lie bed-ridden twice in the last twelve months because of stiff neck and pain in the neck on turnning his face to the right side. He was extremely **devotional to his duties,** so much so that if his work was not over, he used to remain in his office overnight till morning. If things did not go his way, or he was opposed by one, he would get **violently angry.** He was very fond of music, and the only time he could indulge in this luxury was when driving his car to office and back. On the indications: Industrious (SR.630), Mental exertion, agg. (SR461), contradiction intolerant of (SR184), Anger violent (SR.39), Music amel. (SR778), he was given *Aurum met.* 1M one dose. At the end of a fortnight he reported only one episode of headache, with neck pain much better. Another fortnight found him completely relieved in every respect. The prescription was based only on his state of mind and disposition to work hard, with a great sense of responsibility. Rubrics for skin, or headache or stiffness of neck were not looked up at all (Dr. Rajan Sankaran).

Now I will refer briefly to some more cases of Dr. Rajan Sankaran (given in detail in his "Spirit of Homoeopathy"), which in fact have been a source of inspiration to me and many others to practice Homoeopathy on similar lines.

CASE 3 : A woman with total leucoderma came with the history that she had a dark complexion earlier ....She had been to many skin specialists and after trying several therapies they had told her that she had no hope of ever getting back her normal skin colour, and she had better forget about further treatment. She really forgot about it, and came to Dr. Sankaran (after 9 years of leucoderma) with a leucorrhoea which was very acrid and caused intense itching. Dr. Sankaran tried to get details of her case (to elicit peculiar characteristic symptoms of mind and body), but even after talking to her for quite some time he found that he had not got any such symptoms. Then on reflection it occured to him that the lady was very expressive and in her talk there was a lot of humour and joking. Suddenly it struck him that she was expressing the most beautiful symptom viz. "Loquacity with jesting". To this he added "acrid leucorrhoea", "hot patient: and craving for motion in open air. This indicated the remedy *Kali iodatum*. He found in Phatak's Repertory that Kali iod. is listed in the rubric "symmetrical affections". Thus the state of mind (loquacity with jesting) not only cured her leucorrhoea but she got her natural skin colour in course of time. This despite the fact that *Kali iod* is missing in the rubric, "Skin discolouration, white spots."

CASE 4 : A boy of 10 was referred to Dr. Sankaran by a colleague for treatment of a very severe and chronic skin problem. The boy had boils on the extremities which were very painful and itching. For the past few months he could not even sit or stand. He was carried into his consulting room, crying, with boils fulll of pus. The trouble had started since he was 4 months old and all therapies had been tried. The mother reported that the itching was so bad that the boy wanted to tear away his skin. With his hands clenched he shrieked, yelling, "Kill me, I cannot take it. I don't want to live". When itching was too much he said, "Give me a knife; I want to stab my arm". As a child he was very fond of a goddess, but when he despaired of cure he tore the picture of the goddess, saying "what has she done to me?" He could not tolerate even a drop of water,

STATE OF DISPOSITION

did not like bathing, and was thirstless. Rubrics: Impulse to stab his flesh; Cut, mutilate desire to; tear impulse to; Tormented feeling (by goddess), i.e. Delusion, tormented; Delusion, wrong he has suffered; delusion forsaken (deserted) by the goddess on whom he is dependent, he was given *Lyssin*, and he did very well indeed. It is to be noted that Lyssin is not known at all for skin diseases. This was a remarkable case shown on the Video from beginning to end and was received with thunderous applause during the Seminars.

CASE 5 : A case of Dr. B.N.Chakravarty (page 81 of Spirit of Hom.) : A case of pituitary tumour was being taken for operation. The patient, a Minister in West Bengal Govt. developed symptoms of heart failure, every time he was taken to the operation theatre, and he had to be taken home. On the basis of fear causing heart failure, Dr. Chakravarty prescribed *Gelsemium*, Cowardice, anticipatory anxiety, fear of operation, were other symptoms. *Gels.* is not known to have cured tumours, but still it did when it was prescribed on mental symptoms alone.

CASE 6 : Dr. Rajan had a case of Iridocyclitis for whom he prescribed Iodum. Why? Because the patient was hungry every three hours, he had a kind of anxiety that made him walk around. He must walk fast in open air to get rid of his anxiety. He felt extremely hot. He was told that he would become blind if he does not take Cortisone. yet, he got totally well with *Iodum* 200. Dr. Sankaran did not even care to see if *Iodum* has got any eye symptoms.

CASE 7 : A $4^1/_2$ years old girl used to get recurrent episodes of fever with swelling and rigidity of neck with tilting of the head. Diagnosed as Torticollis with acute Tonsillitis. Marked monthly periodicity since the past two years. Neck rigidity associated with severe stomachache and throat infection.

Observation : She was singing and talking to herself;

was very fond of music and dancing. Was very talkative and good at imitation. Very playful, playing with imaginary persons; used to play for hours. Had great imagination. Even in the clinic she was conversing as if with an imaginary person, asking questions and answering them. The parents said that even if the neck is very tender, she is not affected much, unless the fever is very high. "She is very bold and courageous" said her parents, giving various examples. "She was not at all scared of injections and blood collection. If she falls down, she immediately gets up and starts running without crying or complaining. In fact, she has to be constantly watched. We never leave her alone. Once there was a party on the terrace and she was running on the parapet. She jumps from great heights. She runs across the streets inspite of traffic. So, we hold her hand tight, which she resents. She is very restless".

While I was talking with her parents, she quietly slipped away and was found engrossed in her playing. Even when she was sitting on the chair, she was talking with herself and was busy with her game. I talked to her but she was absorbed in her own world. Finally, her parents took away the toy from her hands to compel her to answer my questions. Now, she was quite confused and her answers were unrelated to my questions. Her speech was not clear and the parents had to repeat what she was saying. And when they started talking to me she again went out to play. Her mother told me that she was a slow learner, and her school teacher had even recommended speech therapy for her as her speech was not very clear. Was restless, could not pay attention and was mischievous. Even at school she makes funny noises and faces, not with an intention to make others laugh, but it was a part of her involuntary behaviour. She does not intend to mock or make fun. At home she does not like to drink milk; she pours it into the sink on the sly.

She threatens to vomit if forced to eat or when her

STATE OF DISPOSITION

wishes are not fulfilled. She would break things and become so much aggressive that almost three people are required to calm her down. She loves horror movies and stories of ghosts. F/H eczema and asthma on paternal side; paternal G.M. epilepsy.

Analysis : The courageous part of her nature was superficial but her main symptom was inability to understand danger; absorbed mind, difficult comprehension and concentration, and inability to perform any mental labour. Her talkativeness and mischievousness arose from her retarded mental growth. She was not cunninng. The first rubric I took Ikwas "Runs about in most dangerous places".

Other rubrics : Answers, aversion to (sings, talks, but will not answer questions); Loquacity during which answers no questions. Delirium, romping with children; Chaotic, confused behaviour. courageous. Work, mental aversion to. Foolish behaviour. Speech incoherent. Mistakes in speaking.

She was given AGARICUS 1M, one dose. The frequency and intensity of the attacks started getting less. The torticollis associated with Tonsillitis disappeared. Over a period of one year her attacks of tonsillitis and fever completely stopped. Her performance at school improved and her teachers remarked about the positive change in her state. She needed repetition of *Agar.* 1M on six occasions whenever she had bouts of high fever. She needed *Agar.* 10M after one year, and since then has remained well without further repetition of doses (Dr. Sunil Anand, Bombay).

CASE 8 : A lady, some sixty years of age, looking fit and agile for her age, came in with complaints of itching on the forearms, accompanied by profuse perspiration on the palms alone, even while the rest of her skin remained dry. She was soft spoken and had a well controlled demeanour.

After eliciting the customary information regarding her physical symptoms, I began questioning her on her temperament with a view to fortify her physical traits with the mental picture. What followed was this unusual piece of conversation:

Doctor : How would you describe your temperament?

Patient : Cool tempered.

Doctor : Do you never get angry? **Pt. :** No I don't. Do you get angry doctor? - **Dr. :** Yes, I do - **Pt. :** No, I don't.

Why, doctor do you get angry? - **Dr. :** Yes, , I do. - **Pt. :** If one were to only pause for a moment and think before reacting in anger, it is unlikely that you would ever get angry. **Dr.:** Where is the question of pausing and thinking, because anger is necessarily borne of emotional spontaniety.

Pt. : What is the value of your education if it does not teach you to think, when even with my rather modest education I am able to control and measure my emotional reaction? **Doctor :** Does music interest you? **Pt. :** No, I disapprove of it. **Doctor :** Don't you find music relaxing? **Pt. :** Why does one need external aids for relaxation? If your mind rules over your heart, surely you will find all relaxation within yourself.

One would have ordinarily thought of Sulph. for this philosophical woman, but a search in the Synthetic Repertory with a flicker of hope of finding a fitting remedy, led me to the rubric, "Emotions predominated by intellect" (P.439). Further search through the Repertories gave more rubrics which confirmed *Viola odorata* as the remedy. They are:

Speech, voice low, soft (SR.945) - Music, averse to (SR.778)

Palms moist (Phatak's Rep. 269) - Skin itching and burning (K.1327) Skin, dryness (K.1308) & Phatak 310.

Gave *Viola od.* 30 t.d.s. till visible signs of improvement were seen. Four days later reported improvement. Put on placebo. Two weeks later persistent itching had altogether disappeared. No recurrence to date. (Dr. Parinaz Humranwala, Bombay).

CASE 9 : A four years old child was brought to me for loss of appetite and anaemia with a history of recurrent infection. I observed that he was very upset in my clinic and was constantly muttering 'taking me home'. He had a marked fear of being approached by strangers. He was very careful and cautious not to get injured. The mother said that the child was always scared of falling, even in infancy. These were the important characteristics of his state. So I took the rubrics:

1. Delirium, home wants to go (Syn. Rep. I/215).
2. Fear of injury (S.R. I/506)
3. Fear of falling; child holds on to the mother (S.R.I/500).
4. Fear of being approach (Clarke's Dictionary of M.M.)

From these symptoms I prescribed *Cuprum-aceticum* 1M single dose. To my surprise the child who had not responded to many homoeopathic remedies earlier, showed immediate changes within a week. His appetite improved. He was no longer scared to come to my clinic. He became a healthy child. So, what I treated was not his appetite or anaemia, but his whole state, the real disease in him. There was a relapse of his physical complaints after six months and he had gone into a strong state of Cup.ac. This relapse followed a dental surgery for which he was given a general anaesthesia. I repeated Cup-ac 1M at an interval of 15days and the child's whole state recovered in a month's time. (Dr. Jayesh Shah, Bombay).

CASE 10 : A child of $2^1/_2$ years was suffering from severe constipation right from his birth. He was not passing stool for even four consecutive days. Suppositories and laxatives were of no avail; and he had no appetite. He had been treated previously by a Homoeopathic doctor with Calc. carb (because of fear of lizard, obstinacy, aversion to milk, late talkinng, etc.). This was followed by Tarentula hisp. because the child was sensitive to fast music, he threw things when angry, and was restless. Both the medicines did not help at all.

I gathered the mother's history as follows: She conceived after ten years of marriage at the age of 35, and she was extremely happy, full of joy, throughout the pregnancy.

The father of the child is extremely generous and sympathetic; he wants to do good to others. He is a computer engineer and likes to do creative work.

Nature of child : He was restless; threw things away when angry. Sensitive to music. Has a sharp memory. The parents said (and I also observed) that the child enjoys doing some creative activity.

Analysis of the case : When the mother conceived after ten years, her happiness knew no bounds (more than normal in a pregnant woman), and the child suffered from constipation from birth. So I took the first rubric:

1. Ailments from excessive joy. The other rubrics related to the father and the child, viz.

2. Activity, creative. 3. Memory active. 4. Benevolence, (father). 5. Restlessness. 6. Sensitive to music.

7. Throws things away.

On these indications I prescribed *Coffea cruda* 1M and waited from three weeks. During this period the child had stools at intervals of three days instead of four days earlier. So, I prescribed *Coffea cruda* 10M one dose. From this time onwards, like magic, the constipation had been totally cured, and the appetite is much better. Six months have passed since then and the child continues to do very well.

Conclusion: Not only the mother's state of mind during pregnancy is important, but the father's nature is also equally important while prescribing for a child. (Dr. Sujit Chatterjee, Bombay).

CASE 11 : P.M. 13 years, only son of upper middle class parents; obese, very intelligent has won a gold medal for consistently standing first since class I. Has won numerous prizes in Science and Maths at the National level. Likes to play cricket and chess. Easily gets injured - head or foot (hairline fractures of toes thrice). Intensely shy, never looks into the eye while speaking. Wants to be a computer engineer when older. Sweat profuse esp. on head and upper body. Likes hot bath, cold drinks.

Conscious of being teased about his excess weight and has become fussy about food recently. Occipital headaches often very tense before exams inspite of preparing well. All teachers like him, yet he is afraid of them. Very close to his mother. Always sits bent forward with head down and allows his mother to do all the answering. Various remedies like *Calc. carb.*, *Sil.*, *Tub.*, *Sulph.*, *Arg. nit.* tried but no real results. All would only hold temporarily. The intense shyness and neverousness continued. Recently gave AMBRA 10M one dose. Patient has become leaner and taller, enjoys all games. Sits erect now and answers questions on his own. Indications: Timid, bashful shy. Terrified of strangers, crowd. Frightened of authority (spouse, parent, teacher). Ailments from overwhelming new environment. Dare not express anger due to fear. (Dr. Ranga Krishnan, Madras).

CASE 12 : Sigrid, aged 39. An insecure, timid, worried, gentle woman, mother of three children. She speaks in a low and strained voice. She presents with chronic sinusitis, retronasal catarrh and frequent pharyngalgia, *alternately occurring on one side.* She has suffered from these symptoms for five years. She is tired, feeble and has heavy menses. She feels insecure, unhappy, discouraged, dejected. She describes a *"profound feeling of not being good enough".* *"I am worthless";* she feels excluded from life.

As a child, she had many fears, found it extremely difficult to make friends, was very shy and ashamed, suffered from enuresis. Her father was reserved, aloof, reprimanded her frequently. He had wished for a boy. Her mother was depressive all the time; nevertheless, the daughter still orientates herself far too much towards her.

Lac Caninum 12 x then 200 has given her physical and mental stability during one and a half years' follow up. (Dr. Jutta Gnaiger - Br. H.Jrnl. Jan 1992)

A full volume will be taken up if we list the cases, some very difficult indeed, which have been cured by other doctors in Bombay, (following Dr. Rajan's example) on the basis of the "State of mind and disposition", without caring to check up if the complaint was covered in the relevant sections of the Repertory or materia medica.

How do we explain this phenomenon? :- The successful practice of homoeopathy demands firm acceptance of the tenets, one of which is the concept of vital force, equivalent to "immune force" of the present day. We shall here study the relationship of the vital force with the disease and the place of the state of mind in selecting the curative remedy. This we will do directly from the words and sentences in the "Organon".

"In the healthy condition of man, the spiritual vital

force (autocracy), the dynamis that animates the material body (organism) rule with unbounded away, and retains all the parts of the organism in admirable, harmonious vital operation as regards both sensations and functions". (Aph.9). then, "When a person falls ill, it is only this spiritual vital force...that is primarily deranged by the dynamic influence of a morbific agent inimical to life.... and inclines it to the irregular processes which we call disease"..... (Aph.11). "It is only by their dynamic action on the vital force that remedies are able to re-establish and do actually re-establish health and vital harmony..." (Aph.16) "Man's vital force, when encumbered with a chronic disease which it is unable to overcome by its own powers instinctively, adopts the plan of developing a local malady on some external part solely for this object, that by making and keeping a diseased state this part which is not indispensable to human life, it may thereby silence the internal disease, which otherwise threatens to detroy the vital organs (and to deprive the patient of life)". (Aph.201). "And yet, very little reflection will suffice to convince us that no external malady (not occasioned by some injury...) can arise, persist or even grow worse without some internal cause, without the co-operation of the whole organism which must consequently be in a diseased state...so intimately are all parts of the organism connected together to form an indivisible whole in sensation and functions. No eruption on the lips, no whitlow can occur without previous and simultaneous internal ill-health". (Aph.189). "All true medical treatment of a disease... must, therefore, be directed against the whole". (Ap.190)

"This is confirmed in the most unambiguous manner by experience... every powerful internal medicine immediately after its ingestion causes important changes in the general health... and particularly in the affected external parts... even in a so-called local disease of the most external parts of the body. ... and the changes it produces are most salutary, i.e. the restoration to health of the ENTIRE BODY, along with the disappearance of the external affection - provided the internal remedy directed TOWARDS THE WHOLE STATE was suitably chosen in a homoeopathic sense". (Aph.191)

Now, Hahnemann clearly establishes the link between the deranged vital force which we call disease, and the consequently altered state of mind and disposition. In Aph. 210 he says, "...and in all cases of disease we are called on to cure, the state of the patient's disposition and mind is always altered, and this is to be particularly noted along with the totality of the symptoms.... in order to be able therefrom to treat it homoeopathically with success." (Aph.210). This holds good to such an extent, that the state of the disposition...often chiefly determines the selection of the homoeopathic remedy, as being a decidedly CHARACTERISTIC symptom which can least of all remain concealed from the accuratlely observing physician".(Aph. 211)

Finally, Hahnemann emphasises, "We shall never be able to cure conformably to nature - that is to say, homoeopathically (taking into account the deranged vital force) - if we do not in EVERY CASE of disease, even in such as are acute, observe, along with the other symptoms, those relating to the changes in the state of the mind and disposition - if we do not select.... a disease force (medicine) which in addition to the similarity of its other symptoms to those of the disease, is also capable of producing a SIMILAR STATE OF THE DISPOSITION AND MIND" (Ap.213).

I think that it would be superfluous for me to add any commentary, since the whole idea of what is disease, and how it can be cured by the dynamic force of homoeopathic remedies is crystal clear in Hahnemann's own words.

On a close scrutiny of Aphs. 211, 212, and 213 I was

struck by the fact that in the first two of these aphorisms the altered state of disposition and mind alone is referred to as chiefly determining the selection of the remedy, but Aph.213 stipulates that the medicine selected should be capable of producing a similar state of the disposition and mind, in addition to the similarity of its other symptoms to those of the disease, thus reducing the emphasis on the state of mind. Why so, I began to ponder. I seems to me that it is possible that though Hahnemann had no doubt that the mind and disposition chiefly determine the selection, he felt at the same time that the "other symptoms" of totality should also be considered for confirmation, to make doubly sure and to avoid the possibility of a wrong assessment of the state of mind and disposition. After all, just as each organism is indivisible, so too, the characteristic symptoms (mental and physical) of each remedy run through it like a red thread, and if even one or two most characteristic features of a remedy (like the state of mind) have been identified, the other characteristics of that remedy will follow. This peculiarity if taken advantage of assures us of having identified the correct remedy.

16 Dr. M.L. Sehgal's "Rediscovery of Homoeopathy"

Dr. M.L. Sehgal of Delhi is the founder of what has come to be known as "Dr. Sehgal's School of Revolutionised Homoeopathy" (or "Rediscovery of Homoeopathy"). He regards MIND to be the CENTRE of the body, and therefore the Mind has to be made the basis for selecting the remedy - instead of the Totalityof symptoms comprising symptoms of body and mind. He had found that a specific set of symptoms of the mind - PRESENT, PREDOMINATING AND PRESISTENT - represent the Centre at any given moment. He has also found that when a medicine is prescribed according to the Revolutionish Technique, something in the form of excreta, starts coming out of the body - invariably in every case - which has been found to be leading to permanent cure. Hence the conclusion that certain TOXINS are taken to be the cause of disease. Toxin is a part of the NATURAL MECHANISM of the body. The ordered behaviour of the Toxin is health and the disordered or chaotic behaviour is called ill-health. The homoeopathic medicine just reverts the disordered behaviour of the toxin back to its NATURAL orderly behaviour and thus restores health.

In this technique one observes the way in which the patient presents his case to him (his words, demeanour, manner, expressions and bodily gestures, with anxiety, fear, etc.) He picks out the Present, Prominent and Persistent symptoms and interprets them into Rubrics (called king-pin rubrics) in Kent's Repertory (Mind Section), to arrive at the remedy. Reference to the Materia medica is not necessary. With the help of this new technique the mental symptoms are obtained in a short time. Starting with a small group of students in 1985, Dr. Sehgal today has a large following. As this technique is gaining more and more acceptance from discerning practitioners, it is well worth a serious trail.

A few illustrations of king-pin rubrics and the expressions from which they were drawn will throw some light on the methodology of this unique technique. Thereafter three illustrative cases will be given.

	Expression	Rubric (page No.)
1.	It is for many days now, there is no relief. How long I shall have to wait?	FEAR, extravagance of (45)
2.	Sir, there should be some relief at least to rely upon	Fear, extravagance of
3.	On what basis to wait further?	Fear, extravagance of
4.	Patient is irritable and says for how long I shall have to wait? I am much annoyed with your treatment.	Irritable, pain during (59)
5.	I am at the dead end. No further fight. I am defeated. This is how I feel.	Discouraged. (36)
6.	Somehow I am pulling on, he tells you in an egoistic tone and adds: but if I get medicine it will become easy to do so.	SHREIKING aid for (80)

7. Please do something for me. Call some doctor. I am badly involved. — DELIRIUM, crying for help (18)

8. I was making efforts with the aid of some auxillary means to tide over the phase but it seems I can not depend upon them now. I must call for the regular treatment. — DELUSION, help calling for (27)

9. All life seems to have gone out of me. Limbs become numb and without energy. Everything is as if heading towards stagnation. It becomes so loose and out of co-ordination that ultimately I have to throw my body on something. — TORPOR (89)

10. I want to remain quiet. — QUIET wants to be (70)

11. If I have to think that I have become a burden, I fear that. — FEAR, burden of becoming (43)

12. There is no further way out. — HELPLESSNESS, feeling of (51)

13. I cannot bear it. — IMPATIENCE, pain from (53)

14. I want to be out of this routine. I feel as if I am in a prison. — ENNUI (39)

15. I was expecting some relief. Instead of that, I got headache as an addition to my present misery. — DELUSION, wrong has suffered. (35)

16. If it happens the way I do not want, it angers me. — ANGER, contradiction from (2)

17. I am always worried about my domestic affairs. — CARES, full of, domestic affairs about (10)

18. I have no hope of recovery.	DESPAIR, recovery of (36)
19. Please do not disclose anything about my sickness to anyone.	SECRETIVE (78)
20. Will I be able to go to my work? They say I will have aggravation first?	BUSINESS, talks of (10)
21. Oh, if only I could be saved from the next attack of the disease.	ESCAPE, attempts to (39)
22. I may beat my child and punish him; but he is not bothered about it.	INDIFFERENCE to suffering (55)
23. Whenever someone gives him some hope (light), that his mother will return soon, he laughs.	LIGHT, desire for (62)
24. The child never allows the mother to go out of sight.	CLINGING, to persons. (12)
25. Let me tell you the truth... Actually...	NAKED, wants to be (68)

CASE I treated by Dr. Sehgal's Method where the usual method of Totality of Symptoms had failed.

A lady aged 35 years, with 2 sons, came for intense vaginal itching, which had been present for 1 year, with partial relief from time to time with homoeopathy.

This time she said **very agitatedly** : "Dr. this itching is driving me mad. I can't sleep at night. In the daytime I am constantly shouting at the children, my husband and the servants because of my trouble. The only time I feel better is when I come here and talk of various things, or if I am doing something. I also get a little relief by washing the parts.

I saw my Gynaecologist and she said i had Lichen

Planus. I am thinking of going to a Skin Specialist and maybe I'll have a Pap Smear done.

I am also worried because in a few months we will be transferred and the thought of packing is bothering me. Of course we will have packers to help, but I will have to be around as you can't really trust them. In any case I am very particular about how things should be done."

Then she went on to say that her father who had been widowed recently, had got married to a lady much younger than him, who had a 10 year old daughter. It was obvious from the rest of her conversation that she was more worried about the fact that her share of her father's fortune would be considerably reduced with this new development.

The Rubrics taken were :

Irritability, pains during	S.R.PG.668
Occupation Ameliorates	S.R.PG.790
Anguish, Driving from place to place	S.R.PG. 43
Delusions, thieves	S.R.PG.366
Fastidious	S.R.PG.472
Desires more than she needs	S.R.PG.389
Avarice	S.R.PG.102

The remedy was *Arsenic Alb*. It was given in 1M/3 doses at 10 minutes interval.

She phoned the next morning saying she had slept peacefully for 10 hours, something she had not done for years. More than 6 months have elapsed and she has been well.

CASE II (treated with Revolutionised Homoeopathic technique by Dr. Prabha Patwardhan, M.D. (Paed.), Bombay).

Mr. M.D. 23 years old businessman, came for allergic asthma of two years duration. If he did not take his anti-allergic medicin at bedtime, he would get a blocked nose at night and get an attack of asthma early in the morning for which he would take bronchodilators. He wanted to try homoeopathy. He had tried Nature Cure, Ayurvedic treatment and intensive anti-allergic treatment without much benefit. On various indications I had given him a dose of Sulphur 30; and one week later he said that he felt extremely weak. He felt the medicine was not doing him any good. He felt he should just stay in bed.

RUBRICS :
DELUSION, poor he is
DESPAIR of recovery   PSORINUM
BED, remain in, desires to

Four days later he said he had a very bad attack of asthma, the worst he had ever had. It had started on the first day, had got steadily worse and was very bad on the third day, when he decided to stop Homoeopathy and took some bronchodilators. We had warned about the possibility of an aggravation, but the intensity of the attack made him take allopathy. On the first day of the dose he had felt very calm and tranquil and had slept well for a few hours. After that the attack got worse. This was a good reaction. Mentally he was better and then the physical symptoms had got worse. He was now told that he would be well in a day or two and was given Sac-lac. T.D.S. and to stop allopathy.

Two weeks later: No attacks of asthma. Is keeping very well except for a little nasal discharge. Three weeks later; a little nasal congestion and mild sneezing. Sac-lac. T.D.S Well after 3 days. He needed only one more dose after three weeks, after which there has been no recurrence of the attacks.

CASE III : (Dr. Prabha Patwardhan): I had been treating a 82 year old lady for two years without success.

She had been going down mentally after a hip fracture. She had high blood pressure and had a stroke which left her paralysed on the left side. She is confined to her bed. She stays there with eyes closed, not talking to anyone. Every now and then she starts shouting and then goes back to her state of stupor. She has incontinence of urine and stool and has to be fed forcibly. She does not recognise anyone nor talk to anyone. I had given her remedies like *Baryta carb., Stram, Lach, Sulph.* without any effect.

One of the rubrics Dr. Sehgal explained at a Seminar was, "UNCONSCIOUSNESS, SCREAMING, INTERRUPTED BY" with a single remedy BELLADONNA. Her stuporous state followed by shouting was interpreted as the above rubric and BELL. 30 one dose, with sac-lac. T.D.S. was given. All her allopathic medicines were stopped except a nightly dose of DIAZEPAM.

Four days later a definite improvement was noted. She was alert and remained awake for longer periods. Of course, that meant more shouting. Two weeks later there was no dount that she was improving. She recognised a few people and actually said something. She called out to her son and husband and spoke in three-word sentences. A seemingly hopeless case had shown a miraculous improvement with just a few pills of BELL 30 thanks to the genius of Dr. M.L.Sehgal.

Dr. Patwardhan concludes : In 200 years of Homoeopathy no one has come up with such an imaginative way of looking at rubrics, thus enlarging the horizon and capability of Homoeopathy. To understand Revolutionised Homoeopathy, readers are advised to study the ROH Books Series I to V by Dr. Sehgal in that order.

17 | STATE OF BODY - Effects of latent (Chronic) Infections (Miasms):

Introduction

We have dealt with the importance of understanding the State of Mind and the physical symptoms of the body. There is another aspect of the diseased vital force which has to be taken into account for finding th curative remedy. It is the STATE OF CHRONIC INFECTION which has become latent, and is not easily perceived through manifest symptoms. It is this STATE which puzzled Hahnemann when he found that the best selected remedy had only palliative action instead of helping the rapid, gentle and permanent cure which the truly homoeopathic remedy is expected to bring about. It took Hahnemann twelve years of intensive toil and research to come to the conclusion that what stood in the way of cure in many cases were the three Chronic Miasms, viz., Psora, Sycosis and Syphilis. These conclusions he has succinctly given in his Organon, from Aphorism 72 to 82.

Keen observers and able practitioners of Homoeopathy like Dr. J.H. Allen (Chronic Miasms), Dr. H.A.Roberts (Principles and Art of Cure by Homoeopathy), Mrs. Phyllis Speight (A Comparison of the Chronic Diseases) and Dr. Harimohan Chowdhury (Indications of Miasms) have thrown a good deal of light on the significance and symptomatology of the Chronic Miasms. However, despite all the elucidations given by them, the deep, disturbing and malefic effects of Psora had not been, and could not be, fully and easily grasped to put them into practice - till Dr. Margaret Tyler described the true meaning of the Hydra-headed Psora. Her insightful teachings on this point (given in her lecture/booklet, "Hahnemann's Conception of Chronic Disease, as caused by Parasitic Micro-organisms") quoting massive "evidence" of marvellous cures, must be throughly imbibed by every homoeopath. She asks, "Does Homoeopathy fail us, or do we fail Homoeopathy? Probably, we all of us, limit ourselves to HALF HOMOEOPATHY, and therefore reap only HALF-RESULTS".

Hahnemann said that acute conditions may pass off even without treatment, and that **"Chronic** diseases, only, are the TEST of the genuine healing art, because they do not of themselves pass into health." Every homoeopath has to ask himself how far he is passing this test in his daily practice. A close look at society today, no matter whether rich or poor, will reveal innumerable cases of chronic diseases staring us in the face; diabetes, high blood pressure, kidney disorders, mucuous colitis, tuberculosis, bronchial asthma, mental aberrations, heart attacks, cancer, etc. What is the share of Homoeopathy in preventing, or alleviating, if not curinng, these conditions?

We will take a long step in meeting this challenge if we take up the study of the Chronic Miasms in all earnestness, and do not stop in our endeavour to master this - the other most important "half" side of homoeopathy - till we are able to report successes after successes - as Margaret Tyler did in her time.

I **Understanding THE MIASMS :** We give here what Hahnemann has to teach us:

   1) Chronic diseases owe their origin to a chronic parasitic miasm or germ (micro-organism). They constatntly extend their way notwith standing the

most robust constitution, or the best habits of life (of mind and body) or the most carefully regulated diet.

2) The miasms (read INFECTIONS) may be acute or chronic. Whether acute or chronic, they are parasitic diseases caused by micro-organisms.

3) In both cases the infection takes place in a MOMENT. "If you scarify a rabbit, and take two dabs, (one in each hand) of streptococcus and of iodine, and dab on *one* (iodine) as fast as you can after the other (strepto), you are TOO LATE to prevent infection".

4) All chronic diseases originate and are based on fixed chronic miasms, which enable their parasitical *ramifications* to spread through the human organism, and "grow without end." (Ch. Dis. 1.23).

5) The chronic miasms are semi-vital morbid miasms (infections) of a parasitical nature, which can only be neutralised and annihilated by a *more powerful remedy* producing *analogous* effects." (Ch. Dis.1.53).

6) Gonorrhoea and Syphilis are two Venereal Miasms. They are chronic *parasitic* diseases besed on fixed chronic microorganisms, whose parasitical ramifications spread, e.g. through orchitis which later caused acute gonorrhoeal rheumatism, followed by endocarditis which assumed a malignant type and proved fatal. "The gonococcus was obtained in pure strain from destructive lesions on the mitral valve."

7) Syphilis always follows on the destruction of the chancre by local applications. "Whenever anyone is so impudent as to destroy this vicarious local

symptom, the organism causes the internal syphilis to break out into the venereal disease, since the general venereal disease dwells in the body, and from the first moment of infection it is NO MORE LOCAL.

8) Treatment of the chronic miasms must go on TILL THE CURE is complete, "for the least remains of a germ may eventually reproduce the full disease."

9) Of Syphilis Hahnemann writes: "It never becomes extinct in itself. it increases from year to year, and assumes new and more dangerous symptoms to the end of life." Chronic syphilis will NOT BE CURED with one dose. Hahnemann's great remedy for syphilis is the best preparation of Mercury (Tyler used *Merc. cyn.* with marvellous effect.) He gave it in the 30th potency, but "in cases where a second or third dose (however seldom needed) should be found necessary, a lower potency may be then taken." Tyler suggests: "Besides Mercury, Nitric acid, etc. we have a great remedy for syphilitic conditions in the virus of syphilis : Leuticum (*Syphilinum*), of which night aggravation is a leading indication.

10) The chronic contagion has the peculiar nature of becoming extinct in the body, leaving a SEQUELAE in its train. Many of the chronic infections can enter into a changed, LATENT STATE, and persist as some unrecognised chronic disease. One must RECKON with them if the BEST work is to be done.

II **Miasms (infections) may be either inherited or acquired -**

Thus, a Syphilitic or Gonorrhoeal (venereal) miasm may stem from an indiscretion in the patient's **ancestry,** rather than one committed by himself.

Wm. Boyd, the pathologist, writes (Textbook of Pathology), "Men are not created free and equal but are handicapped from the beginning.... In inherited diseases if the gene is recessive, it may remain dormant for many generations (hundreds of years) before it gets a chance to be free and show it effects." He then gives a long list of diseases of the blood, mentaboilism, skeletal defects, neuromuscular disorders, disorders of skin, of eye, mind, etc. which are all hereditary.

The late Dr. P. Sankaran states in his book "Pathology in Homoeopathy" (Homoeopathic Medical Publishers, 20, Station Raod, Santacruz (W), Bombay, 54): "We have strong reason to think that even the residual effect of various diseases can be transferred to the next generation....the placental barrier does not always protect the child, as German measles, small pox, mumps and influenza have all produced abnormalities .... viruses tend to be transmitted from one generation to another... the latent syphilis can cause thyroiditis and goitre, allergies, dyspepsias, abdominal pain, peritoneal adhesions, chronic ulcerations of mouth, pre-cancerous conditions and even cancer. This is why Paterson, the eminent Bacteriologist says, "Chronic diseases are due to an inherited miasm." Unless these are neutralised, the patient maynot improve".

Fortunately, not every episode of infection gives rise to a miasm. A history of measles (Psoric) as a child does not necessarily imply that the patient has a Measles Miasm. How, then can we decide that a patient has a miasmatic problem, and how do we decide which miasm it is? Firstly, the very fact that the patient suffers from a RECURRENT (chronic) disease, such as ulcerative colitis, or migraine, etc. implies the presence of a miasm (infection), Secondly, one may reasonably suspect the involvement of a chronic Infection if well chosen homoeopathic remedies based on totality of symptoms cease to produce long lasting results after giving initial relief. Of course in coming to a conclusion about the nature of a recurrent disease we have to rule out extraneous factors such as nutritional deficiencies, physical trauma or environmental disturbances.

Dr. J.H. Allen writes (Chronic Miasms, p.135) :"It is often very difficult to see the connecting link between the latent or quiescent state that a miasm assumes and the mysterious processes known as Pathology, that deceive us, or to trace out the lineage from one disease state to another. How short-sighted we are; these latent disease processes are slowly developing day by day, but we do not see the markings or tracings of perhaps psora or some other miasm all the way along. Here is a case of epilepsy, with no apparent cause, coming on in a boy at puberty. Why should this be? Look carefully and you will see a psoric or tubercular diathesis. Again, here is a case of hysteria in a girl of twenty years. She is well developed and to all appearances healthy, but at each menstrual period she suffers in a way that is almost beyond description, violent dysmenorrhoea, extreme pain, spasms, mania with great mental agitation, dysentery and very strange symptoms; and what is the history of such a case? Tubercular, of course; an aunt and an uncle on the father's side died of that disease. It is only a mixed miasm that could give us such a combination of phenomena. Suppose we look over her latent miasmatic symptoms. She has light brown hair that is dry and lusterless, the dental arch is imperfect, the teeth club shaped and irregular, the incisors still show a slight serration, the face is pale, but becomes flushed easily from the least excitement, the eye-lashes are irregular and some of them are imperfectly curved, others stubby and broken, the edges of the lids scaly and red, the hands and feet are cold and clammy, the nails thin and imperfect, split or break easily. All of the above are tubercular or pseudo-psoric symptoms... she has a history of suppressed menses from getting wet in a rainstorm, and all her sufferings have arisen since that time.....A careful analysis of her whole case revealed **Tuberculinum** to be her remedy, which cured the case and she has remained well ever since. Oh, how much there is in treating diseases from a miasmatic standpoint... it means so much to every honest hearted physician who has a desire to carry out the teachings of Hahnemann in order to make perfect cures!"

III **PSORA - the hydra-headed Infections :** It is significant that the indomitable Tyler had the "audacity" to say that "Not one of the great teachers since Hahnemann's day—even Burnett who with his Vaccinosis, came nearest to it—has grasped the true inwardness of Psora", viz. that the cause of disease is the result of infection caused by prasitic micro-organism, a contagion which lies smouldering and becomes latent in the organism." Dr. S.P.Koppikar who unearthed Tyler's unpublished, very carefully prepared, lecture (mentioned earlier) and presented it before an International Congress in Mexico in August, 1980 laments, "What an unfortunate result came out of Kent's observations (Lecture IX on Philosophy) that "Bacteria are the outcome or the results of disease," - whereas Hahnemann repeatedly stressed that diseases are the result of infection caused by the parasitic micro-organism, a contagion which lies smouldering and becomes latent in the organism. Hahnemann talks of Psora as "that immense host of chronic affections", which makes Tyler say that one cannot doubt that "Were Hahnemann alive today, his Chronic parasitic, non-venereal disease (Psora) would long ago have sorted itself out into not one but a DOZEN such."

With the increased knowledge of microbiology today, one can identify a number of INFECTIVE non-venereal diseases which commonly give rise to miasms (smouldering, latent infections). We mention some of them here:

German Measles, Brucellosis, Herpes simplex, Tonsillitis.

Measles, Chicken-pox, Slow virus infecn. Scabies/boils.

Influenza, Parasitic worms, Diphtheria, Mumps.

Scarlet fever, Malaria, Pneumonia, Typhoid.

Tuberculosis, Cancer and AIDS would come under mixed miasms.

We thus see that the Psoric (non-venereal) infection afflicts manking under the names of **different diseases.** It is only when we recognise the origin and nature of these different infections that we will be able to find the curative remedy or remedies for each case. We should remember that latent disease may be extraordinarily quiescent and quite unsuspected. The patient may not be ill, and yet is never well until, as Hahnemann points out, shock, misery, trauma (mental or physical) lowers resistance - and things begin to happen.

IV **Meeting the Challenge :** A few important steps suggest themselves towards helping us to reap the full (not half) benefits of Homoeopathy and to become full Homoeopaths.

1) Probe deeply into the *family history* of each patient- no matter how trivial his presenting complaint, unless it is a very acute condition - the patient's predecessors may have suffered from Tuberculosis, Syphilis, Gonorrhoea or Cancer - going back to atlest three generations. We may find it very difficult to get accurate information, but if we look at whatever data that is presented with a *high degree of Suspicion,* the search may not be in vain.

2) *Personal history* from birth, even going back to in utero, including the "health" (Mental and physical) of the mother, and the information we may get on "Never well since a certain illness" - these are essential.

3) The *constitution* of each patient should be carefully studied, for his disease will be found to be dependent upon some miasmatic basis. The physician should be able to detect the presence of Sycosis for example, in his patient, without a history or gonorrhoea. Let us remember that Phthisis may be headed off before an abscess forms in the lung tissue, if we are familiar with the phenomena of its incipiency. The bond between two miasms can only be broken by a prescription that will *meet the totality of the more active one.* Each miasm has its own phenomena of expression, its times, modalities and order of arrangement. (Chr.M.113)

"The constitutional or chronic miasms may be so latent that no symptoms may mark a deviation from health or show their presence even to one who is skilled in a knowledge of miasmatics. We observe this in growing children and in those of a robust nature in whom strong vitality predominates. The chronic miasms become active in the presence of acute disease (such as the diseases of the children), also at the decline of life, when the vitality of the individual diminishes. It is then that we find tumours, malignant growths and all the pathology that comes through the mixed miasms at the age of decline, from forty years of age and upwards. Such is the history of disease in our works on practice and pathology; the cause always wrapped in mystery and obscurity." (J.H.Allen - 114).

4) Look out for the Miasm in every case :- Failure to recognise the underlying idiosyncracy or chronic miasmatic taint, even in the cure of acute diseases, may prove fatal to the patient; it is one of the difficulties

of the therapeutic art. We must learn to read between the lines, for the symptoms that are often the most prominent and annoying to the patient, are not always the ones to base your prescription upon, and vice versa. An *abnormal symptom* is a sign, mark or indication of a disturbance in the vital force, and its clinical or pathogenetic value is of supreme importance to the physician."

"The physician skilled in anti-miasmatic prescribing **overlooks the foamings upon the surface,** and dips deeper into the case, looking for **prima cause morbi,** and applies a remedieal agent that has a deeper and closer relationship with the perverted life force." (Chr. M.14)

5) "There can be no other "perfection of bond " of psora and syphilis with the life force as is produced through heredity. The tubercular diathesis which is the result of such a union, is one of the profoundest in its depth of action...Specific and malignant, acute, febrile or inflammatory states, as pneumonia, diphtheria, maligna, syphilis, erysipelas phlegmonous, inflammation of the brain, heart, kidney or destructive appendicitis, as a rule, always have the two miasms present. I ALWAYS LOOK OUT FOR THEM IN EVVERY CASE of the above-mentioned diseases." (J.H.Allen, Ch.M.-23)

6) **Which Miasm?**

Once the smoulderinng Infection is identified, we should try to find the "antidote" *analogous to the Causative infection.* It may be a *Nosode* corresponding to the infection, or one of the deep-acting remedies "homoeopathic" to the case. The Nosodes which merit the closest study are : *Medorrhinum, Psorinum, Pyrogen, Secale* (Semivegetable nosode), *Syphilinum, Lyssin, Tuberculinum (Bacillinum), Carcinosinum, Ambra grisea, Anthracinum, Malandrinum, Morbillinum,*

Influenzinum, Diphtherinum, Parotidinum, Typhboidinum, Cholesterinum (A Sarcode).

7) **Iatrogonic Causes :-** In considering these latent infections, we should not ignore iatrogenic factors, in which case Tautopathic remedies have to be used. Tautopathy is a method of curing or removing the bad, or side effects of drugs by iso-intoxication, i.e., curinng by means of the identical harmful agent in potentised form. The deep disturbances of health caused by the heroic dosage of modern medicines have been described by Dr. R.P.Patel in his book, "What is Tautopathy". This is one of the books which every homoeopath must read.

V **Suppression - far-reaching effects :-**

It is within the knowledge of every homoeopath that the vital force in its effort to save the vital organs of the organism from the harmful effects of infections, allows the poisons to express themselves in those parts least harmful, such as through skin eruptions, ulcers, or perspirations, leucorrhoeal discharges, gleet, chancre, warts, etc. Any efforte to eradicate them through local means amounts to suppression, as the result is to drive the poison inside and turn it back on the vital force with serious effects on the general health of the organism. On the contrary, the suffering of the organism is greatly relieved when, under homoeopathic treatment under Hering's Law of cure, some external manifestations of disease present themselves. Therefore, careful enquiry into such suppressions in the life of the patient become imperative.

VI. **Ignore the surface foamings - dig for the deep seated primitive evil:**

When Hahnemann found that even the best selected remedies did not help for long and certain *cases returned again and again*, he concluded that each presentation of the disease did not constitute the disease **in toto,** but was simply an overflowing or a reaction produced in the life force by the presence of some taint, or infection, which he called Psora. The **ostensible disease** was therefore a **mere fragment of a much more deep-seated,** primitive evil, that had taken possession of the whole organism.

Hahnemann concluded from this that we ought not to treat each disease as a separate and completely developed malady; and if we do so, what we do is to drive back the foe, which then repeats its attacks upon the same or some other part under the **false guise of a new phenomena.** This led Hahnemann to insist on the "totality" of symptoms being taken as a therapeutic law.

Unfortunately, the real significance of Totality has been missed by many homoeopaths, who have tended to be satisfied with the surface totality of symptoms of the Mind, the Physical Generals and the symptoms of the Parts. It is necessary to realise that Totality without the image of the Active Disturbing Miasm is an incomplete totality. How do we recognise this Active Disturbing Miasm?

Considering that Chronic Miasms (infections) are mostly latent, quiscent and smouldering in the organism (arising from inheritance or personal history of ailments not fully recovered from or suppressions), every effort must be made to unravel the source and nature of these infections, and to get the image of the Active Disturbing (latent) Miasm.

VII. TRACING THE LINK BETWEEN THE INFECTION (MIASM) AND THE REMEDY"

This is the most crucial question facing the Homoeopath. After all, the ultimate aim is to find the simillimum based on the "Totality" of symptoms which include the symptoms of the Active Disturbing Miasm. The Peculiar characteristics of each miasm given in section XVI are intended to assist the Homoeopath in arriving at the Most Crucial Miasmatic symptoms, out of the LAST APPEARING symptoms, as a basis for arriving at the remedy.

It must be emphasised here that our object is not to "brand" a case as Psoric, Syphilitic, Sycotic or Tubercular, but to identify the peculiar Miasmatic *symptoms* (no matter which miasm) and use them in Case Analysis and search for the remedy. If the Homoeopath gets confused even in this task, **(because it may not be possible in some cases to identify even the so-called most striking symptoms of a Miasm - or even of a remedy),** here is a way to catch the remedy (and through it the Miasm, if at all we must know what Miasm it is)- the remedy that corresponds to the case (totality plus miasm, that is, the miasmatic totality). Based on the (1) Family history, (2, Personal History and (3) Ailments from or.... Never well since a certain illness.... and (4) Suppressions, **identify the Nosode** which is likely to be the remedy for the case; then see if the case has at least a few striking symptoms of that Nosode, to justify its prescription.

ALTERNATIVELY identify three, two or even ONE striking, peculiar symptoms of the case, which are of course **persistent** over a period of time, and see **which nosode** or remedy covers them. That will be the remedy which meets the Present, Active, Disturbing and Dominant Miasm (if you care to name it).

VIII **Tyler on Nosodes :** Margaret Tyler says : "It is recent, rapidly growing experience with the Nosodes of **past acute diseases,** when used for the various conditions that constitute "Old Chronics" that has made one meditate and discuss their possible use in the treatment of Cancer" (Hom. Heritage, Jany. 1992)

Dr. T.K. Moore (H.H. Jany. 1992) adds: "The talented Margaret Tyler.... came to make great play with Nosodes....Recently two cases of antrum infection, were rapidly cured by a few doses of **Streptococcin;** and ear trouble, where measles had been a big feature in past history, has yielded with great improvement on general health and well-being to **Morbillinum.** And now after all these years of dullness and neglect, we are receiving FRESH IMPETUS and are already getting ASTONISHING RESULTS in Heart Disease, in Epilepsy, in rheumatoid cases,even in one case of urgent, hopeless, inoperable CARCINOMA...We have for years been using *Variolinum, Tuberculinum, Leuticum, Medorrhinum* and *Influenzinum.* only *Morbillinum* and some others have till now, not entered into the picture. Tyler has achieved remarkable successes in those patients who have had severe mumps, measles and scarlet fever in early years, and now have obstinate chronic ills, which present COMPLICATED AND CONFUSED pictures to the prescriber.... She has formed the habit of prying into past history for reports of such severe cases of the contagious diseases, whenever difficult, confused, chronic states present themselves. So in the future we shall do well to take notice when told of an old acute illness, **never or tardily recovered from.** Tonsillitis, followed by chorea, then rheumatism, heart damaged in childhood by rheumatic fever, puts in a STRONG PLEA for that mighty remedy STREPTOCOCCIN. Take **the case** of P.K.63 age, male, with gradual loss of vision. No marked generals or particulars. History of very severe "flu" at 18 and again a few years later. A small hook on which to hang a remedy. INFLUENZIN 50M du. Three weeks later: vision greatly improved."

After narrating a number of cures with different Nosodes Dr. Tyler concludes: "One becomes more and more CONVINCED, as one gains in experience, that to CURE it is imperative to give, or to interpose, a dose or two of the most perfect antidote to the ancient malady, viz. its own self, potentised and given in the non-lethal manner of Homoeopathy, only as required, and by the mouth. Burnet. in regard to his especial one, *Tuberculinum* or *Bacillinum*, said emphatically to those who desired to use them *otherwise*, "Hands off." (H.H.Aug. 1983, 373).

Tyler's advice: "We urge the Homoeopathic profession to realise that Nosode treatment.... is homoeopthy and nothing else. Second, to give all the energies of their intelligence to make themselves MASTERS OF THE USE OF NOSODES in their daily practice. They will find a new power for good at their disposal if they do this - only, we must warn them that the work is not exactly as easy as `rolling off a log'.

Dr. D.M.Fobister comments:......"There is a generally accepted principle of homoeopathic prescribing that the remedy which was indicated at the time of acute illness, but was not given, can be effective years later in clearing up an aftermath of illness." (Take as examples : Dunham's famous case of nervous deafness cured by *Mezerium* on the history of suppression of milk-crust 13 years ago. Dr. H.C.Allen's case of impotency cured with *Lac. can* on the history of diphtheria with symptoms of that remedy).

IX **Stop-spot of Remedies :** While managing cases we sometimes find that a remedy which has acted well for some time, has come to a "stop-spot" to use Burnett's expressive description for such a situation. Margaret Tyler throws further light on this phenomenon in her Drug Pictures (p.840). She says that Hahnemann had reached the "stop-spot" of the obvious remedies of present symptoms in chronic diseases; but he had not reached the "stop-spot" of his deductive genius.

Refusing to recognise the "failure of homoeopathy", he dug deeper into the cases and after ten years of labour arrived at the fact that, where more than one disease was in question, remedies homoeopathic to their primary manifestations must be employed, i.e., remedies to suit the miasmatic conditions. Tyler points out that Burnett came up against the stop-spot where one of the "chronic miasms", tubercle, was in question. Such remedies as Aconite, Pulsatilla, Chamomilla and their like "only go up to the tubercular sphere where they come to a spot, and so he began to interpose doses to the tubercle-virus. In the same way he found the stop-spot of the T.B. virus **which acts within its own sphere only.** Other remedies, he says, "are needed for the non—consumptive part of the case".

Hahnemann was already working with other disease-products as remedies, besides *Psorinum*. He designated "the best preparation of Mercury" where the chronicity was based on one or other of the venereal diseases. But here, within their limits, the **most potent of all are the disease-products themselves.** His "isopathic remedies changed by preparation and became "like" or "homoeopathic." She quotes Burnett: "Where vaccinosis is also present, the vaccinosis must be first cured, or the phthisis remains uncured, do what you will."

"Where there is a primary spleen affection that led up to the phthisis, such a case must be approached from the spleen as a starting point, or the treatment fails. When a liver disease underlies the whole maladive state, and phthisis only co-exists with it, the liver malady must first be cured.

"When this state arises from an hereditary

syphilitic **taint** (I say **taint,** not the disease proper), the specific nosode may be required first.

"When the phthisis arises from a cancerous parentage, Bacillinum will not always suffice, until other remedies have prepared the way.

"When the constitution has been damaged by typhoid, by malarialism, by alcoholism, by cinchonism, and so on, all these must be therapeutically reckoned with, or success will not reward our efforts. Wherever, in fact, phthisis co-exists with other diseases or taints of diseases, the **Bacillinum touches the bacillary part of the case ONLY."**

"....I learned the lesson that the pathologic simillimum of a diseases must be administered in high potency and infrequently. Moreover, the worse the case the higher the potency as a rule." (Burnett).

X   A few **outstanding symptoms of some leading Nosodes** are given here is examples; they are not intended to be complete .

(1) **PSORINUM :** Pessimist - hope less despair; Despair of recovery. Offensive discharges, purulent; body smells offensive though well washed.

Feels well the day before the attack.

Chilly - must wear a warm cap even in summer.

Asthma, cough, bronchitis better lying on the back with arms spread out.

Appetite increased at night or in pregnancy.

Itching worse at night, from heat of the bed- sleeplessness.

(2) **SYPHILINUM :** General aggravation of all complaints at NIGHT; feels miserable.

Bone pains aggr. at night; gnawing, sawing pains.

Compulsive (neurotic) checking of things done; washing of hands.

Alcoholism, hereditary tendency to.

Pains increase and decrease gradually.

Leucorrhoea **profuse,** soaks through the napkin, runs down heels.

Ulcerations; succession of abscesses with foul or green pus.

Utter Prostration and debility on awaking in the morning.

Hopeless despair of recovery. Aversion to company.

(3) **MEDORRHINUM"**

General amelioration at the sea and from sea bathing.

History of early heart disease in parents.

Craves Ice; meat fat; oranges; unripe fruit. Craves cold drinks.

Dyspnoea better from assuming the knee-chest position.

Great sensitivity of the soles of feet; cannot walk on them. Uncovers the feet at night; burning feet (Sulph).

Sleeps on the abdomen or in the "knee-chest" position.

Relief with onset of discharges (leucorrhoea, urethral, post-nasal).

Heart, streptococcal infection of -or rheumatoid arthritis (Lyc.Led)

Aggr. daytime; Amel. evening, onset of darkness.

Memory weak; loses thread of conversation.
Painful stiffness of every joint in body - rheumatism.
Intense restlessness and fidgety legs and feet (Zinc).
Intense menstrual colic; terrible bearing down labour like pains; must press feet against support, as in labour.

(4) TUBERCULINUM:

Chronically enlarged tonsils (tubercular family history)

Unreasoning terror in a child at medical examination or with strangers. Uncontrolled tantrums. Shreiking.

Fear of dogs and cats.

Craves cold milk, sweets.

Hyperative, demanding and capricious. Deliberately destructive and malicious; intolerant of contradiction. Indifferent to punishment and reprimand. Head-banging in anger.

Passionate desire to travel. Needs change and excitement.

Emaciation despite eating well (Nat. mur., Iod.).

Allergy to milk and cats.

Worse before storms and change of weather; better on mountains.

Craving for cold milk, smoked meats and bacon, pork, ham.

Long, fine hair on back of children, along the spine.

Recurring chest colds, bronchitis or pneumonia.

Symptoms ever changing; ailments affecting one organ, then another-the lungs, brain, kidneys, liver, stomach, nervous system-Beginning SUDDENLY, ceasing SUDDENLY. (Reverse: *Syphil.*, *Stann.*)

Loquacity during fever.

Aggr. 10 a.m. to 3 p.m.

(5) LYSSIN (Hydrophobinum):

The sight or sound of running water, or pouring water, aggravates all complaints (causes urging for stool, or urine).

Cannot bear the heat of sun (*Gels., Glon., Lach., Nat.mur*).

Impulse to stab himself.

Confusion from dazzling or reflected light, from water or mirror (*Stram*).

Mentally quick and alert; all senses heightened.

Great difficulty in swallowing a morsel, or pills.

Feels the painful sensation of others, as if they are her own.,

Constant spitting ropy frothy saliva.

Very critical and scolding; impatient, violent anger.

Fear of being alone; wants someone next to him all the time.

History of Rabies vaccine in patient or family; or animal bites.

Craving for chocolates; or "strange" things during pregnancy.

Inclination to be rude, to abuse, to bite and strike, reckless.

Sexual desire abnormal. Vagina very sensitive, rendering coition very painful.

Thirst with inability to swallow. Severe constriction of throat prevents swallowing - even speech is difficult.

Bluish discolouration of wounds.

(6) CARCINOSIN:

H/O fright, unhappiness, anticipation.

Fastidious (*Ars., Nux., Anac.*)

Obstinacy and love of travel (*Tub.*)

Amel. at sea (*Med.*)

Sleep in knee-elbow position, first year in infancy. (Older children: *Tub., Phos., Sep., Lyc., Calc.ph., Med.*)

H/O T.B., Diabetes, pernicious anaemia, or a combination of all of these.

Blue sclerotics; cafe au lait complexion - Multiple moles.

H/O inflammatory illnesses (whooping cough, pneumonia); a long list of them.

When children have had an unusually large number of acute infections.

Dancing love of, and of music.

Craving: Salt, fat, eggs, spicy food; milk, fruits; chocolate.

Averse: Fat.

Sympathetic - Loves the excitement of thunderstorms. (*Sep.*)

H/O Diabetes in both parents (Foubister)

XI **NEVER WELL SINCE** .... or Ailments suffered from in the dim past which have or could have left a strong morbid effect on the organism - and the corresponding Nosodes/Remedies:-

Measles	Morbillinum
	Kali Chloratum
Tuberculosis ..	Tuberculinum
	or
	Bacillinum
Septic conditions, blood poisoning, Puerperal fever not treated properly	Pyrogenium
Typhoid	Typhoidinum
Tonsillitis	Streptococcin
Syphilis	Syphilinum
Small-pox	Variolinum
	Thuja,
	Silicea.

Small-pox-		Prophylactic: Maland.
Malignant ulceration, sloughing; Felon, Carbuncle-gangrenous; with HORRIBLE BURNINNG PAINS	-	Anthracinum.
Vaccination	...	Thuja, Sil., Malandrinum.
Dog-bite or Anti-rabies injection		Lyssin, Belladonna
Diphtheria	...	Diphtherinum, Lac can.
Mumps or its Matastasis	...	Parotidinum
Influenza	...	Influenzinum or tuberculinum
Gonorrhoea	...	Medorrhinum
Footsweat, suppressed (Foul)	...	Silicea
Herpes Zoster	...	Variolinum, Ars. alb., Ran. bulb., Mezerium.
German Measles	-	Rubella
Scarlatina	-	Scarlatinum

XII **USING NOSODES :** Dr. E.Underhill., M.D. wrote in his article in Hom. Recorder, 1929 (Hom.Her.May 1990) : "Allow me to emphasise the point stressed by Kent, Allen, Felger and others that the nosodes are to be prescribed on the symptoms and not for the disease of which the particular nosode is a product. When you prescribe let it be always upon the ESSENTIAL SYMPTOMS similarly existing between the patient and his remedy. This important rule of practice need not hinder us from observing that *Tuberculinum* is frequently indicated in obstinate and confused cases where there is a FAMILY HISTORY of tuberculosis, and the *Medorrhinum* is often indicated in conditions undoubtedly sycotic in origin." .....I have seen *Syphilinum* do apparently nothing in known syphilitic cases both inherited and acquired. But I have also seen it work wonders in other cases, perhaps syphilitic perhaps not, where the SYMPTOMS OF THE PATIENT

MATCH THOSE OF THE REMEDY. In the discussion on this paper Dr. Farrington said: "I liked the stand Dr. Underhill has taken that we should prescribe these remedies SYMPTOMATICALLY and NOT give them merely on the supposition of a preceding miasm.

Dr. H.C.Allen in his classical work, "Materia Medica of the Nosodes", writing under Medorrhinum says: "The nosode is just as effective in homoeopathic practice, prescribed strictly on its symptomatological basis as any other remedy. If the symptoms of the patient call for this remedy it should prescribed with the same confidence as any other in the Materia Medica, entirely irrespective of the sycotic history in the case. Like EVERY OTHER NOSODE, it should be **prescribed according to its strict indicaitions,** just as we prescribe *Arsenic, Opium* or *Sulph.* irrespective of origin or the diagnosis."

Intercurrent Remedy? Dr. F.E.Gladwin, M.D., a student of Kent, says in her article "The Intercurrent Remedy", (Hom. Recorder Jany.1929): "When the `indicated remedy' did not act I gave the `Intercurrent' and expected the miracle, but the `Intercurrent' did not act either....This happened many times. One day I asked Kent about this and he said: "We older men have fallen into the habit of leaving the word "seemingly" out of that phrase "seemingly indicated namely fails", Then I saw that the so-called 'indicated remedy' was only seemingly so and was not the indicated remedy at all, and the so-called INTERCURRENT REMEDY WAS THE TRULY INDICATED REMEDY. The truly indicated remedy had been masqueradinng under the name of `intercurrent remedy'.

XIII **Treat the latest, most outstanding totality first - till cure;** "We can never tell how the life force may react under the right remedy or the proper potency;

that belongs to the mysterious law or action and reaction...The reaction depends upon the nature and stage of suppression, and upon the bond of the miasmatic element on the life force... As the sycotic discharge lessens, the secondary eruption or the syphilitic roseolic flush becomes more prominent upon the chest. In a MIXED CASE AS ONE MIASM DISAPPEARS OR IS CURED, the latent one becomes suddenly active.

Dr. H.A. Roberts expresses the same point thus. "In treating the combined stigmata, the most outstanding must be treated first... taking the most outstanding symptom totality. After that is eradicated or considerably lessened, the next most potent dyscrasia AS IT EXPRESSES ITSELF IN THE SYMPTOMATOLOGY, must be treated, UNTIL THIS TOO IS ERADICATED. The treatment should continue in this way, EACH TIME treating the most dominant stigma as EXPRESSED by the OUTWARD MANIFESTATIONS, until cure is attained.... It is not always necessary, if a remedy be carefully selected, to zigzag a chronic case towards cure. Nevertheless, our treatment must ALWAYS BE BASED UPON THE TOTALITY OF THE SYMPTOMS AS THEY MANIFEST THEMSELVES. The homoeopathic physician has the power to forestall the destructive processes of many chronic diseases.... and this gives us the opportunity and the privilege of correcting these devastinng scourges."

Dr. J.H. allen emphatically states (Chr. Miasms II-107) :"In no instance should the MENTAL PHENOMENA OF the MIASMS be overlooked in the selection of the remedy covering the case, for the MENTAL SHOULD PREDOMINATE over the physical always, and each of the chronic miasms has its own morbid mental peculiarity. Much care should be taken to watch them in the progress of cure."

XIV **Potencies :** "Only the higher Potencies have proved satisfactory in these cases of suppression; the lower potencies seldom accomplish the work, or have the desired effect. A suppressed disease seems to have such a complete bond with the life force, that **only the higher potencies reach down** deep enough to sever the bond. It is only when we see these facts demonstrated in practice that we can come to a true realisation of it... However, especially in sensitive organisms or those easily affected, the lower potencies are to be used, such as the 30th, 200th and the 1000th.

XV **Re-establishment of suppressed discharges:**

As soon as old gonorrhoeal or gleety discharge is reestablished, the other symptoms, whatever they may be (even of the severest type or character) usually subside... even scirrhus or abnormal growths, no longer increase in size... affected joints often greatly deformed, resume their normal condition; in short the disease disappears under the use of the higher potencies." The writer has seen all these things take place. (J.H.Allen: Ch. D. II-126-7)

XVI **Characteristics of Miasms:**

In order to be able to see the connecting link between the functional or pathological disorder and the latent, quiescent chronic infection (miasm), we must acquire a comprehensive knowledge of the peculiar characteristics of these miasms. Dr. J.H. Allen says, "Each miasm has its own peculiar history, its physiological expressions, its mental phenonena, its aggravations of time and circumstances, its secondary and tertiary menifestations upon mucous surfaces or upon the skin". All these espects have been clearly elucidated by Dr. H.A. Roberts, Dr. J.H.Allen, Dr. Phyllis Speight, Dr. Harimohan Choudhary.

Indications of Miasms : A few of the most important peculiar indications of the Chronic Miasms given below will help us to recognise each of them. " The very earmarks of the various stigmata (miasms) show their respective characters."

The **Psora** itches and appears unclean, unwashed.

The **Syphilitic** ulcerates, and the body structure is changed.

The **sycotic** infiltrates and is corroded by its discharges.

Perspiration - Psora : better from perspiration.

Syphilitic patients are aggravated by perspiration.

Time : Psora : repeated attacks of fearfulness during the DAY with or without pain.

Syphilis : All symptoms are worse at NIGHT.

Organs & Tissues affected:

Psora : Spends its force when suppressed, upon the nervous system, largely, or upon nerve centres, often producing nervous and mental phenomena of a serious character, all ameliorated when an eruption is thrown upon the skin.

Syphilis : Flies to the meninges of the brain and to the brain itself, to the larynx, throat in general, eyes, bones and periosteum.

Sycosis : Attacks the internal organs, esp. the pelvic and sexual organs in the worst specific forms of inflammation producing hypertrophies, abscesses, cystic degeration, mucuous cysts, etc., and when thrown upon the brain it produces headaches, severe acute mania, central insanity, moral degeneracy, dishonesty, etc.

STATE OF BODY

Thought process :

Psora : The psoric patient is bright, active, quick in movement. A chronic grumbler, never satisfied with his condition. Full of fears; fears darkness, to be alone, fears an ordinary ailment, and thinks that something serious will happen, Restless in thought, feeling and hence in action. His thoughts run so fast, that he is never at a losss for words. Delusions of all kinds.

Syphilis : Dull, stupid and specially stubborn, sullen, morose and usually suspicious. Depressed, keeps troubles to himself; a close mouthed fellow. All quickness of thought is gone; gradual incapacity for understanding things - this makes him morose. (Psora opposite). Has to read a piece over and over again; reads but cannot retain it. Forgets what he is about to utter. (Sometimes observed in Tubercular children). Reasoning power is slow.

Sycosis : Fits of anger. So suspicious, he dare not trust himself. Must go back and repeat what he has done or said. Suspicious that he will be misunderstood, which leads to the worst forms of jealousy of his friends. Tendency to make a SECRET OF everything. Cannot trust others. Quarrelsome; tendency to harm others, harm animals. produces the worst forms of cruelty, cunning, deceit, worst form of mania. Mean and selfish, a liar and vicious scoundrel, devoid of all love and affection; mean and selfish. Makes a beast of man. Self-condemnation. Mental conditions are all better by return of old ulcers, discharges, warts, etc.

MIND : Psora makes the mind overactive; **Sycosis** malactive; and **Syphilis** under-active.

Psora is quick; *Sycosis* is bad, and *Syphilis* is slow.

Psora is intelligent, *Sycosis* is mischievous and *Syphilis* is idotic.

DESIRES & AVERSIONS - they stand high in therapeutic value as they are basic miasmatic symptoms, next in importance only to perverted mental phenomena in disease.

Psora : Craves sweets, acids and sour things; unusual things in pregnancy. Loves sweets, sugar, candies and syrup like hot foods.

Pseudo-Psora : (Tubercular) : Extremists; like hot or really cold things. Long for indigestible things, chalk, lime, slate pencils etc. Will eat salt alone from the dish, more than all the family put together. Longing for stimulants, beer, wines. Craves potatoes and meat.

Sycosis: Craves beer though it is not advisable. Wines aggr. Should take sparingly of meat. Gouty conditions cannot digest nuts. Meat promotes the uric acid and gouty diathesis.

Syphilis : Likes cold foods.

Pathology : Pure Psora does not produce any STRUCTURAL changes; Psora does produce FUNCTIONAL changes. The psoric patient always fears that he will die from heart trouble; but he lives long and "produces income for the physician" (R). He is the victim of so many unpleasant sensations that he requires much attention. It is the SYCOTIC AND SYPHILITIC heart patients who die and that suddenly, and without warning. The psora heart conditions are much influenced by strong emotions, grief, fear and so on. He is found constantly taking his own pulse. (HAR).

XVII Illustrative cases :

1. A striking case of a woman who hasn't had a normal movement of the bowel for over 20 years...She was going to the hospital... and was willing to be opened

to find out what was the matter. She said, "If I could feel as good during the day as I do at night, I would be alright. From the time the sun comes up until it goes down, I feel badly." I didn't ask her any more questions. I gave her *Medorrhinum*. She wrote to me two weeks later: Had some pain for four hours, and is now having normal bowel movements. (Dr. Krichbaum).

2. A 11 year old boy in bed with fever of 103° F; room stifling, but a wool muffler wrapped around his head; pale, dirty skin, drenched in fetid sweat, slight thin discharge from ear which could be smelled on entering the room. Pain if head is raised on a pillow. History of frequent running of the ear since scarlet fever at four years of age. *Psorinum* 10M one does. Fever dropped in two hours. ear discharged violently for a week. Chilliness, sweat and odour gone. No ear discharge for ten months, when it became necessary to repeat the dose. (Dr. Elizabeth Hubbard).

3. A farmer brought her twelve years old daughter carrying her in his arms, requesting that her limbs be restored for use.When asked for the cause and how long she was in this state, the father said that she had an attack of measles about a year ago, after which she was paralysed while her health was otherwise good. The patient could kneel with ease, but could not stand. The trouble was therefore, not in the hip-joint, but in the knee-joint. She had no pain and could, while sitting move her limbs at pleasure. On account of the measles which had preceded, I gave her *alium Chloratum* 6, in pellets, three to be taken dry on the tongue three times a day. I was not a little surprised and astonished to see her, four weeks later, with her father, standing and walkinng on her feet. She had felt a change in her legs as early as the sixth day after commencing treatment. (Dr. C. Assem, Perior - H.H. March, 1990)

4. Was asked to see a lady suffering from a very evident attack of influenza. Under treatment the acute symptoms subsided within a short time. But there remained a condition of fever with very little else in the way of symptoms and all my efforts to help failed towards real improvement. At last one day, the patient complained of a little pain in the right foot; she had not thought it worth mentioning. On looking at the foot I found it red, swollen, shiny and very tender. The mystery was solved! I was dealing with a case of gout and did not know it - until it "kicked" me in the eye. Yet I might have guessed it before. The patient was an extremely gouty lady and the INFLUENZA HAD STIRRED THE GOUT into action. *Urtica urens* Q (Dr. Burnett's pathologic simillimum of acute gout), and the foot was nearly normal in twenty four hours. (Dr. J.H.Clarke on "The value of Accurate Diagn.") Clarke adds: "When the nosological diagnosis enables you to hit your pathologic simillimum, do it by all means and you will score every time."

5. Dr. Clarke writes : In May 1904 I was written to about Mr. D. Two years earlier he had a bad attack of influenza. The melancholic state, which followed and lasted for months, passed off. The following year (August) he got wet through in pouring rain. Before the wetting he had felt pain in the right foot, which was felt more and more after the wetting. It kept him awake at night at last it bacame so bad as to cripple. Of the three well-known consultants one opined it was neuritis and the other two felt that it was tumour of the spinal cord. Inspite of negative x-ray and spinal puncture, the lumbo-dorsal spine was unroofed and the canal thoroughly explored, and the tumour was missing still. The patient was sent home as nothing more could be done for the "wasting of the spinal marrow". At this stage Dr. Clarke was approached through letter with the history: A healthy man

previously; had typhoid at 15; twice vaccinated. Mother died of tumour in the throat and father in an accident. Patient liable to bronchial colds in cold weather. The patient suffered from shooting pain right through the soles of the feet up to the knees. Feet swollen and discoloured. Locomotor power of both feet was lost. Pain was worse after sitting up awhile. Was better in hot weather. Damp had no effect. During intense pain the urine was reddish.

How to solve this puzzle? On which line of similarity to open the attack ? - The trauma of operation, or the classical symptom similarity, or the proximate cause of wetting; but the pain started before the wetting! I traced the essential cause to the attack of influenza which had made such profound impression on Mr. D. some eighteen months before, Now in the course of my materia medica labours I was struck with the similarity of the PATHOGENESIS of *Tuberculinum kochii* to the late effects of influenza, as I had observed them in practice. I had also seen the bad effects of influenza on phthisical patients. I therefore concluded that Tuberculin of Koch might form the PATHOLOGIC SIMILIMUM of late influenza effects, in the same way as *Thuja* is of Vaccinosis and *Sulph. Psorinum* etc. of Psora. The law of similars was true here as elsewere. Tub. koch will not cure all cases - of course not. Every rule in homoeopathy must be used WITH BRAINS, and Homoeopathy has always a reserve when our first effort fails us. Thus, *Tub. koch* 100 was given in three powders out of 24 night and morning. The patient made a steady recovery with occasional repetition of doses, and with symptomatic simillimum (*Plumbum acet.* 100 and *Alumen* 100) following.

Whatever may be said of other methods of hitting the simillimum the importance of finding the

PATHOLOGIC SIMILLIMUM is sometimes of the vary first order. To do this we must diagnose the pathology of the case, and must have the works in which you can find the pathologic similimum. (Dr. J.H.Clarke).

6. **Bright's Disease :** A young woman suffering from Bright's diseases was in hospital and at the end of two months was declared incurable. Because of abnormal brightness of eyes and dialated pupils *Belladonna* had helped her greatly, but only temporarily, As her condition was pitiable, I made a thorough examination of the cause of her trouble and learned that it dated from a large abscess, the result of a lanced and badly cared for felon on the thumb of left hand. Soon after this the swelling of the feet and face commenced. Urine showed an enormous amount of albumen and a variety of casts. Feet and legs terribly swollen; much puffiness of face. Concluded, here was a suitable case in all respects to give *Pyrogen* a trial. So *Pyrogen* CM was given. After a frightful aggravation, with groaning and moaning and piteous crying, I was determined to make no change in the remedy or dose or habit of life, she began to improve after two months, and was discharged as cured after three months. I have omitted to mention that the headache was accompanied with profuse bleeding at the nose and nausea and vomiting. Dr. Bell cured a case of blood poisoninng with Pyrogen and I was so impressed with its power. He gave me a vial with an urgent request to use it if I had a dissecting wound. It has proved a life saver in several cases of malignant typhoid fever. (Dr. Thomas M.Dillingham - Hom. Heritage, Feb. 1983)

7. **Chorea :** Girl of 9, gramacing and twisting; temperature 99.6; heart irregular with impure first sound at apex. *Hyos*, failed to help. *Nat.mur* did not cure. But she had pneumonia twice and once broncho-pneumonia. So she got a dose of *Pneumo-coccin* 200 and soon cleared up. Better than for years, said the mother a

month later. Never needed a second dose. (Tyler - H.H. March, 1983)

8. **Post-influenzal Epilepsy :** Fits ever since influenza 12 months ago. Severe fits several times a week, with enuresis. Also fits with very violent temper... Was given Influenzin 200 three doses six hours apart. She needed no other medicine. Report: No more fits.

9. **Chronic Measles benefited by its Nosode :** a boy of 12 brought for heart. Had measles at 7 years old; haemorrhagic, coughing blood from lungs, bright red and frothy. Temperature was then 105". He was very ill. Cannot run fast. Breathless on stairs or when hurrying; gets very pale if tired. Heart very irregular. No really illuminnating symptoms except a great fear of the sea. Was given *Morbillinum* in 20,30 and 200 on three successive days. Recent report : He is strong and well. The school doctor found heart greatly improved. Has never looked back. (Tyler - H.H.March, 1983).

10. I have always found that in cases of prolapsus or any malposition of the uterus and its appendages, our female sex is put to mental disturbances - nay, sometimes they turn maniacs. I can cite instances to show that there is a vital connection between the disorders of female parts and the balance of the mind. I had a case of a full fledged insane female whom I cured with *Pyrogen* 10M, the only hint I got was that two years before, she had an attack of Puerperal fever which was badly handled, and though the patient recovered she was not cured; it was a zigzag recovery only. This history suggested to me Pyrogen, the only symptom calling for it was inveterate constipation; only a few balls of intensely offensive odour. She was cured as soon as a pitch dark and offensive lochia was discharged following the administration of my remedy. (Dr. N.Ghatak - H.H. Feb. 1989).

11. A boy of 12 was in the collapse stage of a severe attack of cholera with clear symptoms of Carb. veg. But he did not respond even from 200 to 50M potencies. At this stage one symptom of Medorrhinum (Allen's Keynotes) came to my mind, i.e. **state of collapse**. When questioned the boy's father admitted an attack of gonorrhoea years ago. One dose of Med. 200 dramatically brought him from the jaws of death. (Dr. J.M. Kanjilal - Ind. Jr. of Hom. - Oct. 1981)

18 Remedy Response - Second Prescription Managemenement of the Case

Every prescription made after one that has acted is known as the second Prescription - even if it is the nth time that it is made. The second prescription is a most onerous task because it has to take into account a number of factors, especially assessment of the type of response which the previous prescription has evoked.

There are mainly five types of responses to a prescription:

(1) Aggravation of symptoms (2) Aggravation of the disease, (3) Amelioration of the complaint (4) No change (5) Return of old symptoms. It is important to know how these responses arise, becuase only then will we be able to tackle them suitably. Hahnemann states (Aph. 156) that it is almost impossible that medicine and disease should correspond as accurately in their symptoms as two triangles with equal sides and equal angles. The result is that when the curative power (the drug plus the right potency to match the disease force) is inappropriate, a pronounced increase in the suffering (aggravation) follows. Therefore, if there is an aggravation of symptoms, we have to decide what is the cause and what action should follow. Dr. Kent has beautifully summarised these responses in his "Lectures on Homoeopathic Philosophy". They are given here in a condensed form.

1. "If the aggravation is long, with a decline of the

patient's strength, the case is incurable and can only be palliated. In such cases begin with 30th or 200th potency and observe whether the aggravation is going to be too deep or too prolonged.

2. If the aggravation is long, with a slow improvement, all will be well if the remedy is not soon repeated.

3. If the aggravation is quick, short and strong, with rapid improvement of the patient, this is the best result.

4. If the remedy and the potency administered are quite suitable, in exact proportion to the quality of the sick-making force, then do we have a cure without aggravation. This is the highest order of cure in acute affections.

5. If we have an immediate amelioration, followed soon by an aggravation, either the remedy was only superficial and could only act as a palliative or the patient is incurable. Re-examine the case and find out whether the remedy covered the whole case; let the patient wait through grievous suffering for the new picture.

6. If too short an amelioration follows a pronounced aggravation, it will prove incurable. It means that there are structural changes and the organs are in a precarious condition.

7. If a full time amelioration of symptoms occurs without any increase in the patient's strength, he will prove to be too weak for restoration to health. There are latent organic conditions which prevent improvement beyond a certain stage.

8. If the patient develops symptoms of the remedy given, without improvement in his disease symptoms, the case is a hard one to treat even for an experienced

homoeopath. As he proves everything given in higher potencies, go back to the 30th or 200th.

9. If old symptoms appear with aggravation, you may wait; you need study no more. you have the remedy. Cure is taking place according to Hering's Laws of Driection of Cure. Let the medicine alone. However, if the old symptoms come back to stay, then repetition of the dose is often necessary.

10. If there is a transference of symptoms form circumference (periphery) to Centre (e.g. from knees to heart), antidote the remedy AT ONCE.

Let us go though the practical application of these observations.

1) When the patient is improving after the prescription, it is quite good. But it is important to know whether it is the improvement of the general state or of a few symptoms. The real improvement which is a cause for satisfaction is when it is an improvement in the general condition, a feeling of well-being. If every remedy palliates the suffering, but does not bring about the cure (general well-being), doubt arise if it is a curable case - or whether we have touched the real depth, the submerged miasmatic state of the case.

2) What do we do when the patient is improving? WE MUST WAIT - HANDS OFF, so long as the curative impulse continues. To repeat the medicine, or to change the remedy just because there has been a slight change in the symptoms is to "Crush your work" as Margaret Tyler puts it. "All things oppose haste in prescribing ... especially with the second prescription than the first...many a life has been saved by waiting and waiting. For example: A little girl suffering from diphtheria was in a very bad state .... After a long study the child received one dose of *Lyco.* cm. which cleared out all the exudation... but did not touch the larynx.

I dare not tell you how long I watched that child before I saw an indication for the second remedy... I waited until the poor child was threatening dissolution, when I saw a little tough, yellow mucus in the mouth; *Kali bich.cm.* one dose cleared the larynnx in one day". (Kent's M. writings)

3) **HOW LONG** should we wait? We will know if we know the **reasons** for waiting:

(a) If the patient reports a sense of well being (even if his local symptoms may possibly be unchanged or worse): WAIT. The remedy is acting and it is "criminal" to interfere with its action.

(b) If the symptoms are aggravated with new symptoms of the remedy prescribed, it is clear that the remedy is overacting - and it should be let alone to exhaust its overaction.

(c) If there is a return of old symptoms (according to Hering's Laws of Direction of Cure) the old symptoms recur in the reverse order of their first appearance, this curative process demands that its shall not be interfered with.

(d) If some of the old symptoms remain and new ones appear, we should wait until the new symptoms become stable, definite and clear. Only then will they be a guide to the remedy now needed.

(e) If the local symptoms are apprently worse (cough with easy expectoration, increase in eruptions with increase in exudation) and at the SAME TIME the patient is not worse, it is the natural development of the disease and curative in its effect.

(f) If the amelioration of a few symptoms is accompanied by a decline in the patient's strength and cheer, the medicine has acted unfavourably. If it is a chronic disease cure is doubtful.

(g) If comparatively harmless symptoms have become

dangerous (from a synovitis to a carditis), a speedy antidote is required.

(4) "In cases where a low potency had been administered in frequently repeated doses, I have observed that some time must elapse before a perfect action will follow in higher potency; but where the dose had not been repeated after its action was first observed, the new and higher potency will act promptly". (Kent's Minor Writings p.234)

(5) "When the symptoms come back unchanged after prudent waiting, the selection was correct, but if the same potency fails to act, a higher one will generally do so quite promptly, as did the lower one at first. When the **picture comes back changed** only by the absence of some one or more symptoms, and NO NEW SYMPTOMS, the remedy should never be changed until a STILL HIGHER POTENCY has been fully tested. - No harm can come if a single dose of the medicine has been allowed to exhaust its curative powers; it is even negligence not to do just the thing. (K.M.W.234).

(6) When the present remedy has done all it is capable of doing through a range of potencies, going up to the highest, then the time has come for the next prescription. **The LAST APPEARING SYMPTOM shall be the guide to the next remedy.** This is so whenever the image has been permitted to settle by watching and waiting for the shaping of the returning symptom-picture. Caution : If the last appearing symptom is an old symptom on its way to final departure, no medicine to be thought of (Hering's Law).

Acute Exacerbations of a chronic state : When acute exacerbations recur again and again (e.g.bronchitis), and every time we are able to palliate, we have to recognise the predisposition to recurrent attacks in some chronic infection. We have to allow the true image of the sickness to express itself through several of the exacerbations taken as a whole. A single paroxysm does not fully express the totality, but several must be grouped and the true image will be discovered. If the acute disease be uncomplicated with a miasm, the indicated remedy will wipe it out *"cito, tuto et jucunde"*. (K.M.W. 235)

Latent period of action : When we have selected the remedy with all due care and study we should have FAITH in its power. The length of time it may take to act is not so important, and "wait" is the only safe thing to do. Kent says, the finest curative action I ever observed was begun sixty days after the administration of the single dose. The curative action may begin as late as a long-acting drug can take to produce symptoms on the healthy body.

This brings to my mind an article titled "Latent Period of Remedial Action" by Dr. S.P. Koppikar (Homoeopathic Heritage, Dec. 1991). He cites the case of a friend, during his college days, who was down with Pleurisy. Dr. S.N. Sengupta was called to see him and he prescribed *Kali bich* 200 one dose and plenty of placebos. When he reported to Dr. Sengupta that there was no progress he asked "Are there any new symptoms?" - No. "Is he worse?" - No. Then more placebos. This went on four times, and suddenly on the fourteenth day, the temperature touched normal, the patient had fine sleep and in one day was perfectly well. On this Dr. Sengupta remarked, "The dose must take its time to cure , you know!" Dr. Koppikar has cited another case, that of his uncle who had Osteo-arthritis of both shoulders which not even the best homoeopathic treatment ould help. One day, in despair he took *Aur-met* CM, one dose, led by Dr. Clarke's comment on the "profound solvent action on the tissues and new growths". For six long weeks there was no change, neither for better or for worse. But in the seventh week, one day he felt a bit easier in the morning and within three days, the entire stiffness, pain and every vestige of Osteoarthritis disappeared. Again, a case of caries of the clavicle not improved after two operations, was cured with *Silicea* CM single dose when, after three months of patient waiting, the sequestrum came out and ended the trouble. Dr. Koppikar writes about more cases of warts cured in outstation patients (who could not come frequently) than City patients who continuously pester and don't allow time for the remedies to act. In his essay on Typhoid Fever. P.P.Wells has coined a new phrase for this period of no apparent action as the period of "Latent Medication". Such protracted delay in seeing the effects of well-selected remedies is observed in chronic pathology or as after-effects of acute viral infections. They call for more than common firmness and nerve on the part of the physician.

Relationship of Remedies to be kept in mind:

In managing a chronic sickness the remedy that conforms to an acute experience of the illness is worth knowing, as very often its chronic may be just the one that conforms to the symptoms. For example, when Puls. is of great service but only for a short time, the symptoms may now point to its chronic Silicea. (K.M.W.239). The second prescription must be one that has a friendly relation to the last one. Similarly remedies having inimical relationship, like *Causticum* and *Phos.*, or *Apis* and *Rhus tox* should not be given one after the other.

When a succession of remedies is required: It sometimes happens that a case presents symptoms calling for two or more competing remedies, and the patient may thus need more than one remedy (Aph. 170). It will not do in such cases to give both those remedies together or in alternation. The case should be re-examined afresh and a differennt remedy found for the latest symptoms. This involves a process of zig-zagging the case to a cure, either because of lack of knowledge of our remedies or because the case does not unfold fully and clearly before us when we first consider it. Some call this a process of removing layers or of peeling the onion. There is another reason for this, viz. the removal of one miasmatic condition may bring to the surface the submerged miasm. We cannot expect to eradicate any stigma or contagion with a single remedy- and a succession of remedies becomes necessary.

That we need not look down upon "Zig-zagging" is shown by the following observations of Dr. Wesselhoeft:

> "A remedy cleans as much as it can and no more. Then, in the second examination, that is, the second picture we get, we will have to be as careful as with the original examination. Many years ago, when quite a young man, and soon after the provings of Apis were published, I had the good fortune to cure a young lady, who at every menstrual nisus was insane, with this remedy. I reported the case to Dr. Hering and Dr. Lippe, and asked them what I should have done if Apis had not come to our knowledge. Dr. Lippe replied: "You would probably have "zig-zagged" her into health by Pulsatilla, Sulphur and Graphites, which would have taken longer and you would have probably got there in a year instead of two months".

Zig-zagging because of "stop-point" of Remedies :
We had occasion to learn earlier about the "Stop-point" of remedies from Burnett and Margaret Tyler. It automatically follows that we have to zig-zag when we are confronted with the "Stop-point" of a remedy. Dr. Sarabhai Kapadia's views on this subject are relevant. He says, "The curative range of a remedy is the same as its pathogenetic range. Burnett

termed it "the stop point of a remedy" beyond which it cannot cure. The "Stop-point" of medicinal action can never be determined by a study of apparent totality of symptoms. Every drug has its own limitation of curative range which has got to be worked out only in the clinical field. A drug cannot cure something which it cannot cause. *Aconite, Bell.* have no application in typhoid even if the apparent totality of symptoms indicates it. Nor can you cure Tuberculosis with *Bryonia*. Determination of the curative range cannot be done in the proving. It has to be judged in careful clinical work, or in the case of poisonous drugs, by inference from cases of poisoning. (Ind. Jrl. of H. Med. Jul-sep. 1976).

Take the new (latest) symptoms for the second and subsequent prescriptions : Erastus Case quotes Aph. 169 to support his second prescription. When symptoms remain after the first prescription has exhausted its action, viz. "a more appropriate homoeopathic remedy must be selected for the set of symptoms as they appear, on a NEW INSPECTION". Hering makes the same point in his "Analytical Repertory of the symptoms of the Mind" (p.24)

> "In all chronic and lingering cases the symptoms appearing last, even though they may appear insignificant, are always the most important in regard to the selection of the drug. The oldest are of least importance. All symptoms in between have to be arranged according to the order of their appearance".

Dr. E.Case draws a lesson from a serious case of Sarcoma in a three year old child, and stresses that this lesson should be prominently borne in mind:"

> "At one period an attempt was made to go at once to the root of chronic disease by giving the constitutional remedy first, even when not fully

indicated. That prescription was apt to raise such a turbulent storm of symptoms that it was difficult, often impossible, to control the patient. The conclusion was soon reached that the correct method is to **prescribe for the present conditions,** bearing in mind as especially important the latest symptoms that have arisen; then to follow the case backward, step by step, removing the ailments in the reverse order of their first appearance. Finally, the constitutional remedy becomes clearly indicated, and it will complete the cure gently and safely".

When the pains and sufferings cannot be distinctly perceived:

Dr. E. Case says that we sometimes meet a condition in acute diseases where the patient feels himself very ill, but the symptoms are indistinct owing to a depressed state of the sensibility, so that he has no clear symptoms of his sufferings. In a case of this nature, Opium in a high potency will remove the torpor of the nervous system, and then the symptoms of the disease develop themselves plainly in the reaction of the organism. (Footnote to Aph.183). I have known an instance of this in typhoid fever, where no clear disease image could be obtained. Opium 30 in a few hours restored the vitality of the patient so that the remedy which restored health was easily found.

19 CONCLUSIONS AND PLAN FOR ACTION

After having studied what the various master prescribers have said on the approaches they adopted to satisfy the principle of "totality of symptoms" in order to find the simillimum, it is time we now summarise the kernel of their teachings. A careful study of what all of them have said will take us to the conclusion that it is the "striking, singular, uncommon and peculiar (characteristic) signs and symptoms of the case of disease which should chiefly and almost solely be kept in view" for the purpose in view-irrespective of whether these singular, unusual and peculiar symptoms which characterise the patient (not the disease) pertain to his mind and disposition, or his bodily functions, his personal or family history of infection or even the peculiar symptoms of pathology. Hahnemann even went to the extent of saying (Aph.164) that the "small number" of such uncommon and peculiarly distinctive symptoms in the best selected remedy is no obstacle to the cure. In the early days of Homoeopathy when there were no detailed Repertories, the masters had to wade through the vast symptomatology of remedies. It is in this situation that Guernsey and others hit upon the brilliant idea of "Key-notes" which could guide one to the remedy. Guided by the keynote one had only to check up if that remedy had the other characteristics also of the case in hand. The only condition for a keynote to be used legitimately in a case is that it should not lead to a remedy whose generals do not conform with the case. In other words, the test whether a remedy selected on the basis of keynote is the true similliar lies in the fact that it should also cover at least some of the other leading characteristics of the patient.

Let us turn to what Dr. Erastus case says about the symptoms that guide, in his book "Some Clinical Experiences". Dr. Case (1847-1918) was a truly gifted clinician with a rare ability to clearly perceive his patients and prescribe the curative remedy. His book contains 212 clinical reports of ninety different diseases treated mostly with the highest potencies in a single dose of remedies (sometimes rare) selected on the basis of Peculiar characteristics, the Keynotes. Dr. Case describes his method of arriving at his conclusions, thus :

> "I follow **two methods** in my work : **One** is to pick out the **uncommon or peculiar** symptoms and find the remedies that have them; then hunt up the one that has the **rest of the case** in its pathogenesis. The **other way** is to take the locations and corner the remedy down by the **modalities** usually by means of the Boenninghausen Slips".

In another place Dr. Case observes:"Now we see why our earlier attempts with the repertory failed of the best results. We were placing the absolute (i.e. common) and general symptoms alongside the *characteristics* as of equal value, instead of giving the former a secondary place, and **using them to confirm the choice of the remedy made from the characteristic symptoms**..... It may be urged that a characteristic symptom cannot be found in every case; but surely no two persons are just alike in form and feature, and the differences in the constitution, and in the disturbance of the physical economy in disease, are so great that **individual peculiarities are always present.** Our success will be determined in great measure by our acuteness of observation in recognising the peculiarities of the patient, and our skill in adapting to them the appropriate medicine."

Dr. Case lays down fourl Rules for the choice of the remedy:

(1) **Other things being equal, give the preference to a mental symptoms rather than to a bodily one.** Example : A case of Lyc. which may be arrived at by the rather long process of elimination if several physical genneral symptoms are taken, but *Lyco.* could be arrived at straight away when the peculiar weakness of mind (weakness of memory) was given the highest value.

(2) **If there is no peculiar mental symptom, use the most peculiar bodily one** - Example : A boy of 12 years, a haemophilic, who would bleed to death from a slight cut unless pressure was applied, is the patient. Six weeks ago he received a bruise upon the left buttock. The blood escaped into the cellular tissues until the thigh was enormously distended. He has been lying in bed awaiting the absorption of the blood. He is deeply jaundiced with itching skin. Bowels constipated and stools composed of small, white, round balls. Profuse haemorrhage with the urine, both fresh and coagulated blood. Stitches between the scapulae upon every attempt to swallow, so that he abstains from food and drink. Since a chill yesterday he has high fever with sleepless, restlessness and white coated tongue.

The symptoms of skin, stool and urine and knee have been present several days. One would scarcely expect to suffer **pain between the shoulders from the action of deglutition.** So far as ascertained, that symptom belongs to only one remedy. *Rhus Toxicodendron.* The jaundiced skin and white stools are pathological, and neither belongs to Rhus. The haemorrhagic diathesis, haematuria and white swelling of the knee do not belong to it. Although one symptom only calls strongly for Rhus, it is SO **VERY PECULIAR** THAT IT **OUTWEIGHS** ALL THE OTHERS COMBINED. He received a powder of *Rhus* 1m dry on the tongue every two hours, four doses in all. The interscapular pain was relieved immediately, the urine was free from blood on the following day; on the second day the bowels moved naturally with stool of normal colour and character; in ten days he was in as good health as he ever enjoyed.

(3) **A common symptom by concomitance, may become characteristic** Example : A dry, tickling, **spasmodic cough at night, relieved by sitting up,** pointed to *Hyos.* which cured immediately.

(4) **In subsequent prescriptions, when the same remedy is not indicated, follow the latest symptoms which have appeared. —**

Example: A complicated case suggested Ars., Lyc., and *Nux vom.* to antidote drugging with allopathic medicines. Six days after *Nux-V.* 30 the patient presented symptoms of Lyc. which cured the symptoms and brought back symptoms of asthma (suppressed) nine years back. *Ars.* cured fully.

I feel that there could not be a better, and more authoritative, summary than this of the principles for the choice of the CRUCIAL symptoms viz. that the choice should depend upon the nature of the MOST PECULIAR symptoms we have been able to elicit in each individual case, and at each stage.

How to identify the uncommon, peculiar symptoms: This is a question of crucial importance. Naturally, as Kent has so clearly put it, all the symptoms of the patient **minus** those pertaining to the disease he is sufferinng from, are the uncommon symptoms which characterise the patient. It is these uncommon, unusual and peculiar symptoms which guide us easily to the remedy.

The problem of identifying peculiar symptoms is not different from that of identifying a person (even a well known actor) or a certain make of a Car. The eyes do not see, nor the ears hear (perceive, recognise) what the mind does not know. Therefore, the solution to the problem of identifying anything lies in knowing it beforehand. We should therefore, know (recollect and discuss with friends) as large a number of peculiar symptoms as possible - at least the most typical of them to begin with. Now, let us get down to the task of knowing the peculiar symptoms.

Mental symptoms, or symptoms of Mind and Disposition" :

Although Hahnemann has stressed the signal importance of these, we can imagine how difficult it was to know them in the early days of Homoeopathy. To begin with, Boenninghausen did not choose to extract as many of them from the Materia Medica for presenting them in the **Therapeutic Pocket Book,** as did Kent in his Repertory. With the publication of the Synthetic Repertory we see more and more cases being treated with the mental symptoms than was possible before. After all, the Homoeopath is like an Artist who, though a master of the **techniques** would be handicapped if he does not have the **best working tools,** so essential for putting his techniques into practice. (Many more symptoms of the mind have yet to be incorporated into our repertories, and this task will continue (as heretofore) as clinical confimations and contributions from discerning, efficient practitioners are brought on record).

What is the source from which we can easily master the mental symptoms? It is observed that it is easier to know them from the Repertory, with the Rubrics and sub-rubrics alphabetically arranged, rather than from the Materia Medica directly. We must therefore try to become thorough masters of the various rubrics. If one wants to know how the various rubrics are arrived at after interpreting the patient's experessions of his complaints, the relevant chapter in the "Spirit of Homoeopathy" and the small book, "Probing the Mind" by this writer would help.

It sometimes happens that one faintly recollects a rubric but finds it difficult to locate it readily in the Repertory. This problem is easily solved by a reference to "The Word Index of Expanded Repertory of Mind symptoms" by Dr. H.L. Chitkara.

Physical Generals : The next class of guiding symptoms are the Physical Generals. These relate to the man as a whole and not to his Parts, which latter are called Particulars. We have already seen earlier that Particulars can even be ignored unless they are characterised (qualified) by striking location, sensations, modalities or concomitants. Physical Generals fall under a number of sub-classifications. A few of the most leading symptoms of this category are given in Appendix "A". They must be committed to memory, if we are to "Catch" the characteristic symptom when it is being narrated by the patient.

Peculiar, uncommon (i.e. unusual), even strange (which cannot be explained) symptoms have been discussed before. Whenever a patient refers to a strange symptom we should take a special note of it and should not consider any effort too great to track down the remedy which has it. Dr. Erastus Case noted down every single peculiar symptom which came to his notice while studying cases or the materia medica. He thus compiled a large number of them and "learned more keynotes in one year than in the preceeding five years". It is obvious that this compilation was the secret of his astounding success even with rare remedies. A thorough mastery of these symptoms will therefore amply repay all the efforts in studying them. However, as these are too numerous to easily remember, a few *typical* ones are given in Appenndix "B". The reader would do well to have these at his finger-tips so that he does not pass them by when the patient spontaneously expresses them while narrating his complaint. In suitable cases we may even have to pointedly ask the patient about any of them. For example, a patient having acute pain in her abdomen would not have spontaneously given us the vital unusual symptom, "the pain comes gradually and also subsides gradually" if we had not asked her about it. Correct prescription of *Stannum* would have been unthinkable without this characteristic.

Causation : The importance of causation of complaints (Ailments from, or ailments ever since an event) cannot be under-estimated. The cause may be proximate causing an acute attack, such as diarrhoea, vomiting, headache, sleeplessness etc. The cause may be grief, shock, pecumary loss in businness, disappointment, disappointed love, insult, suppressed anger, wounded honour, etc. which are all given under the heading, "Ailments from" in the Synthetic Repertory Vol. I. The cause may be proximate (recent) or remote (fundamental or a chronic infection - Miasm). The fundamental cause may be indicated by the symptoms in the present or it may be a submerged state with no presenting symptoms to guide us to the remedy. In the latter case we shall have to try to bring out the Cause by discreet enquiries and a "high degree of suspicion". In any case, it is absolutely necessary to delve into aetiology in every case in view of its great importance in the selection of the remedy.

Concomitants : We have already dealt with their importance in the choice of the remedy, under chapter 5.

PLAN FOR ACTION

Case Taking : The reader may well ask, "Does not the large number of "Mental, Physical General and Peculiar" symptoms given in appendices "A" and "B" (not to mention many more given in Allen's Keynotes, etc.) be taken the need for an extensive case taking session?" No, it does not. We are not going to ask the patient about each of these points. The correct method of case taking requires that the physician encourages the patient to tell everything about himself, his emotional and mental make-up, the life-time effects of certain events and sufferings he may have undergone, his chief complaint, etc. The physican should take careful notes of the patient's statements and underline those parts which are expressed spontaneously, with force and clarity. After he has finished, the doctor may ask for clarification of those statements which are not clear or complete, or ask for additional information which he may not have voluntiered. The patient may take 60% of the whole time involved in taking the case, the doctor takes 25% of the time for interrogation and the remaining 15% is taken up for analysing the case and identifying the most crucial, indispensable, peculiar symptoms.

In case-taking the patient (and his attendants) have to be guided at the outset to throw light on every little detail about the patient and his complaint, especially those which he may *regard as strange, unusual or even funny*. When the patient is narrating his case, we should be particularly attentive (sharp witted) to note any peculiar or unusual symptoms of mind and body. Remember : The more successful we are in eliciting such peculiar symptoms which have their counterpart or similar in the materia medica, the easier it is to select the curative remedy. In other words, we have to seize upon any remark, even casually expressed or in a flash, which connotes a peculiar symptom. Peculiar symptoms have to be largely gleaned from the patient's demeanour, manners, tone of speech, etc. If at any stage he hesitates to speak out, we may suspect that he does so as he feels that we may laugh at his peculiar symptom. We should remove his fear and encourage him to unhesitatingly describe what he feels. In case he has not covered any specific points in Appendix "B" (which we consider essential), we may ask for information about them, of course without putting "leading questions" which can be answered with a "yes" or "no".

The doctor is in the position of a commander at the Army Headquarters. Unless the Commander is thoroughly familiar with the topography, the terrain, the rapid-flowing rivers, the deep valleys and the precipitous hill-slopes as well as the strategic passes, etc. in the battle front, he will not be able to spot the weak points in the enemy's defence system and **determine the few most vulnerable points for attack.** In the same way, a good knowledge of the various types of peculiar, striking and unusual symptoms (mental or physical) on the part of the doctor will enable him to immediately identify any peculiar symptom which the patient expresses. Without this knowledge, even the most peculiar and highly useful symptom will pass unnoticed. It is for this reason it is said that without a good knowledge of the materia medica (especially the Peculiar, uncommon symptoms of remedies), the case taking suffers - and how can we hope to find the curative remedy without a well-taken case? As Dr. D.M.Foubister said: "What is wanted is not a mass of symptoms, but a picture of the individual reaction in proper focus, with the **very few definite** symptoms in the foreground. One of the remedies which covers the **few salient features** will usually be found to cover all the rest."

Analysis of the case : After taking the case in detail, the prescriber has to decide, on the basis of the data before him:

1. Whether the patient's health has been affected following some event (mental or physical) which has left a **"lifetime effect"** on him. This includes the long-term, sub-merged latent effects of some chronic infection (Miasm) arising from family history or history of his personal illnesses.

2. Whether the patient has "never been well since" (Ailments from) an identifiable cusative factor-including suppression of a skin affection, or emotional shock, grief, disappointment, fright or serious attacks of jaundice, typhoid, tuberculosis surgery, diphtheria, measles, etc.

3. Whether the physician has been able to clearly understand the patient's state of mind and disposition - and if not, whether he has at least identified the outstanding symptoms of the mind and disposition.

4. Whether he has been able to elicit at least a few strange, rare, unusual and peculiar symptoms.

5. Whether he has noted the outstanding Physical Generals with their Modalities etc.

6. Finally, whether he has identified at least some Particular symptoms complete with their location, sensation, modalities, causations and concomitants.

Now, analyse the data under the above six heads carefully and arising from these approaches make a list of the most peculiar, uncommon striking and strange symptoms (mental or physical)- the FEW CRUCIAL symptoms, which can help you to arrive at the simillimum.

Take these striking, outstanding symptoms through one or both of these two filters:

CONCLUSIONS AND PLAN FOR ACTION 143

1. The Minimum Syndrome of the Maximum Value (three-legged stool) filter - the remedy being confirmed by the "Genius" of Remedies; or

2. The Repertorial filter. For doing this take one or two MOST Peculiar and outstanding symptoms (Rubrics) in the Repertory as the PIVOTAL points, and set out in a chart the two and three marks Remedies common to both of them, with their respective marks under each remedy against the rubric concerned. Carry this process down to cover the remaining CHARACTERISTIC symptoms (of mind and body). Study the emerging remedies for their correspondence with the case, to arrive at the simillimum.

Example : (taking only 3 marks remedies)

	Hyos.	Lach.	Lil-t.	Sulp.	Verat.	Zinc.
Religious (KR.71) (Pivotal Rubric)	3	3	3	3	3	3
Vertigo, closing eyes on (KR.98)	-	3	-	-	-	1
Sleepless, waking after (KR.1254)	-	3	-	2	-	1
Warm air agg.	-	3	-	2	-	-
		12/4				

Reference to the "Genius" of remedies for the Mentals and Physical Generals, and to the Materia Medica for other symptoms will confirm Lachesis as the remedy. The prescriber will develop the art of this type of analysis and the ability to choose the curative remedy as he studies more and more the cases successfully treated by able prescribers, and constantly learns from his own experiences as well.

Posology.

We shall turn to Dr. Erastus Case again for his succinct advice. "There is no known philosophy regarding the potency to be used, that is authoritative. I have no doubt that cures have been made by all dynamisations, from the mother tincture to the very highest that have been prepared. Each must follow the course to which study and experience shall lead him. I have been led to adopt the following rules:

Rule I. Give the higher potencies to those accustomed to the low or to allopathic treatment.

Rule II. To those accustomed to high potencies, give still higher, or much lower; that is, change the potency for the patient.

Rule III. After improvement stops, change the potency if the same remedy is indicated.

Repetition of the dose

Rule IV. In cases with a well marked exacerbation give a dose at the time of, or immediately after an attack. Disregard of this rule has often caused an aggravation. (For example, it would be correct to give a dose after every stool in diarrhoea, and unsafe to give" a dose every three hours").

Rule V. Repeat the dose until an effect is produced, then STOP.

Rule VI. Never repeat a remedy so long as improvement continues, even if it is slow. Impatience has many times spoiled the case for me.

Dr. J.T. Kent on Posology : In any discussion of Potencies and Repetition of the Dose we cannnot ignore Kent's advice, as he was a master in every sense of the word. He says:

CONCLUSIONS AND PLAN FOR ACTION 145

"The perverters of truth claim that the self-same agent will cure in any dose or any potency. My statement is that the simillimum, the **curative power or force** is not essentially the curative **drug.** The simillimum may be found in Aconite 200 where Aconite 3x has failed. Then Aconite is the curative agent but not the simillimum, but Aconite 200 is the simillimum. Where Aconite tincutre cures, and cures permanently, I believe it does so because it is the simillimum. I have recently seen Ars. 200 fail in a case so clearly indicating Ars. that a tyro could not fail to see it, and the same 200 is known to be genuine and has for years served well; the 8,000th of Jenichen cured promptly. *The remedy was Arsenicum, but the simillimum was Ars. 8m....* I admit it is seldom necessary to be so exclusive in finding the curative power, but that it does sometimes occur I am more than convinced".

"It is much more satisfactory to use a very high attenuation of any drug believed to represent the curative power in a single dose. It is the safest and surest way to avoid a mistake. If the remedy acts, it is so permanent and almost sure to be the simillimum. **If it does not act,** there is no harm done and a lower potency may be selected. If a lower potency is selected and repeated, as often has to be, the overaction spoils the case and sometimes precludes the possibility of a cure. (Minor Writings, page 82).

"The physician who knows how to use the various potencies has ten times the advantage of the one that always uses one potency, no matter what the potency is". (M.W.640)

"Many chronic cases will require a series of carefully selected remedies to effect a cure, if the remedy is only **partially similar;** but the ideal in prescribing is to find the remedy similar enough to hold the case through a full series to the highest.....The patient can feel the medicine when it is acting properly". (M.W.641)

"To suit all degrees of sensitivity in chronic diseases the physician must have at his command his deep-acting medicines in the 30th, 200, 1000. 10m, 50m, cm. and mm. potencies. (M.W.439).

"I observed sharp aggravation when beginning with the CM. but seldom observed aggravation when beginning low in relation to the sensitiveness of my patient's nature. Of late years, *I always begin lower and gradually go higher*, and thereby avoid shocking even the very sensitive women and children. (M.W. 676).

"In my judgement the selection of the best potency is a matter of experience and observation and not as yet a matter of law." (M.W.474).

"An axiom: When the symptoms change, the remedy must be discontinued, as it ceases to be homoeopathic... if continued it may be detrimental..... It is unsafe for the beginner to indulge the desire to repeat too much - it should always be restrained". (M.W.440)

"The nature of the disease makes a difference; patients who have heart disease, or who are suffering from phthisis are apt to have their sufferings increased and the end hastened by the highest potencies; they do better under 30th or 200th. Sometimes very sensitive persons will do well on a high potency if they have been prepared for it by the use of lower one". (M.W.450).

For more detailed and excellent guidance on Posology, readers are requested to study the chapter 'Homoeopathic Posology' in Stuart Closes "Genius of Homoeopathy."

20. THE BEST TEST OF A HOMOEOPATH

Kent said (Heritage, Mar. 89) : (we abbreviate) : Learn well the symptoms of every disease and all disease ultimates - so that you can perceive what symptoms are **not common;** symptoms which are not common must be UNCOMMON AND PREDICATED (in genneral or particular) of the patient. These must be foremost in guiding to the remedy.. When this method is mastered, prescribing becomes easy, with experience.... If we fail to cure sick people we are not homoeopathicians.

The curing of sick people permanently, gently and quickly is the first and BEST TEST of a homoeopathician. If the remedy is properly chosen and administered in typhoid fever, how soon should the patient recover? Every homoeopath should be willing to have himself measured by his answer.

Looking back over thirty years, I can answer the question better than a young man. My cases of continued fever with prostration, tympanitic abdomen and sordes on the teeth recovered inside of two weeks in the first ten years of my homoeopathic practice. In the last twenty years they have all been aborted in seven to ten days. Not one has continued to progress according to the usual course of the disease; therefore, not one could be proved to be typhoid by the Widal test.

The homoeopathician will never have a case that will stand the eighth day test, therefore, according to modern science, he will never have a typhoid.

Hahnemann says that all acute disease should be aborted. Why should we not expect to do this if Hahnemann did so a hundren years ago? Why call ourselves Homoeopathicians if we cannot do as well as Hahnemann did? Why not offer this as the test of our ABILITY AND SKILL ... or CEASE to call ourselves homoeopathicians? (These views of Kent were pronounced in 1912, four years before this lamented death).

Incurable Cases? "The same law applies in curable and incurable cases, and it is very essential in curable cases that no narcotic nor hypnotic nor sedative should be used, for the reason that these cloud the whole conndition.... In incurable cases, or seemingly incurable cases, we must not put a limitation on the possibilities of the similar remedy, for in many seemingly incurable conditions the simillimum will so completely meet the situation as to obliterate the symptomatology of disease and the pathology, and will restore the patient to health. (H.A. Roberts Priniciples 168).

Appendix 'A'
Physical Generals.

Here are a few leading Physical General Symptoms which every practitioner must be thoroughly familiar with

(1) Thermal modality : Better or worse from heat or cold air, or weather or season (as applied to the whole person). Also from the heat of sun, hot or cold bathing, draft of air.

(2) Time modality - General and particular - Exact time of the onset or peak of complaints; or morning, afternoon, evening, before or after midnight.

(3) Periodicity of complaints - Alternate days, weekly, yearly, summer, winter, etc.

(4) Modalities of Circumstances, such as Aggravation or Amelioration (General or Particular) — whether the patient or his particular complaint is better or worse Before, or During or After each of the following Circumstances:

(i) Eating (ii) Drinking (iii) Cold or warm drinks or food (iv) Stool (iv) Urination (vi) Coition (vii) Lying on back, on left side, or on right side, knee-chest position or on abdomen (viii) Sleep (ix) Menses (x) Exertion, mental or physical (xi) Hanging down of limbs or keeping them elevated. (xii) Looking up or down or sideways (xiii) Touch, even slight. (xiv) Pressure, simple or hard (xv) Lying with head high or low (xvi) Nature of sleep or loss of sleep (xvii) Loss of vital fluids: Blood, semen, leucorrhoea (xviii) Stooping or standing straight. (xix) Overlifting (xx) Motion, slow or fast, or at perfect rest (motionless) (xxi) Strong odours (xxii) Light or darkness (xxiii) Thunderstorms (xxiv) Noise, sudden (xxv) Rubbing (or magnetism as some call it)

(5) Appetite and thirst : Whether normal, extreme or wanting. when and under what circumstances.

(6) Cravings for and Aversions to (or Aggravation from) certain items of food or drink. They are all listed in Vol. II of the synthetic Repertory.

(7) Nature of sleep :disturbed; sleepiness; sleeplessness before or after midnight, or after certain hours; sleepless after waking up for any reason; sleepless from thoughts or activity of mind (brooding, planning); sleep Unrefreshing in the morning. (Also position in sleep).

(8) Dreams which are more or less repeated; vivid, frightful, pleasant, etc.

(9) Sexual impulse (desire strong or weak); Complaints of sexual function.

(10) Menstrual disorders; leucorrhoea.

(11) Perspiration - whether partial (hands, palms, feet, scalp, etc.); Profuse or scanty. Whether it stains or stiffens the linen. Whether offensive; cold and clammy.

(12) Motion of one arm and one leg.

(13) Painlessness of complaints usually painful.

(14) Paralysis one-sided, or of single parts.

(15) Heat, flushes of, with profuse perspiration.

APPENDIX 151

(16) Marked, severe, sensations of pain such as Burning, Cutting, Jerking, Throbbing, Stitching, Sore or bruised etc. with their modalities and locations.

(17) Emaciation, general of the whole person, or of single parts: Cervical, Wrist, Extremities. Compare Atrophy.

(18) Sensations as if flesh were loose; or floating in air; as if legs are not his own, etc. (Look up H.A. Roberts' "Sensations as if" or those given in J.H. Clarke's "Dictionary of Practical Materia Medica").

(19) Effects of Moon Phases (Full Moon or New Moon) on the complaints.

(20) Disproportion between Pulse and Temperature.

Appendix 'B'
Peculiar Symptoms.

Here are a few of the most typically strange, peculiar and uncommon (unusual) symptoms which the practitioner should enquire into in every case, to ensure that no significannt aspect of the case is overlooked.

(1) **Side of body affected** - right, left or diagonal, or from right to left or left to right; or alternating sides.

(2) **Direction or Extension of the symptoms** - downward, outward, upward, radiating. In other words, the part from which the pains extend and the parts to which they do so (given at the end of the main rubrics of pains in Kent's Repertory). The "Directions" will be found in Boger - Boenninghausen's Repertory, page 892.

(3) **Alternating states** - Diarrhoea alternating with constipation. Eczema with asthma; physical complaints with mental, Numbness of foot alternating with numbness of hands (K. 1042)

(4) **Manner of oneset and exit** of symptoms (K.1377): Whether increasing gradually and decreasing slowly; or increasing suddenly and decreasing suddenly, etc.

(5) **Area of pain :** Whether in a spot (K.1385 - B.Boenn. 923); or radiating in all directions, or whether they are not in a fixed place and are wandering from one area to another (K.1389).

(6) **Discharges** : Sweat, expectoration, urine, coryza, leucorrhoea, stool,, menstrual flow, etc. -their consistency, odour, colour, acridity (burning) or blandness; mucous or bloody.

(7) **Discolouration** of face, lips, around the mouth, Linea nasalis, circumscribed, etc. bluish, pale, cyanotic, red (flushed), - under various connditions like during headache, chill, menses, cough, excitement, toothache or from fright or shock.

(8) **Hanging down** of limb aggravates or elevating it ameliorates the pains (K.1009).

(9) **Nausea** at the thought or sight or smell of food. (K.507).

(10) **Sensations as if** : when these "sensations as if" are clearly expressed by the **patient himself,** and when the remedy indicated by these "sensations" matches with the other characteristics of the patient, they assume decisive importance. These "sensations" more correctly represent sensory perceptions, while if they arise from feelings, they may more approapriately be termed as delusions. It is worth consulting H.A. Roberts' "Sensations as if" whenever we come across them in a patient. (See para (18) in Appendix 'A')

Appendix 'C'
Important Aphorisms from the 'Organon'

Some of the important Aphorisms in the 'Organon' are given here, as briefly as possible, in order to focus attention on the most important points contained in each of them. Readers would do well to ruminate and ponder deeply over them to grasp their full significance as guides in their practice.

Aph. 6: The unprejudiced observer - well aware of the futility of transcendental speculations which can receive no confirmation from experience - ... takes note of nothing in every individual disease, except the changes in the health of the body and of the mind (morbid phenomena, accidents, symptoms) which can be perceived externally by means of the senses....he notices only the deviations from the former healthy state... all these perceptible signs represent the disease in its whole extent, that is, together they form the true and only conceivable protrait of the disease.

Aph. 7 : .... It must be the symptoms alone by which the disease demands and points to the remedy suited to relieve it and more over, the totality of these symptoms, **of this outwardly reflected picture of the internal essence of the disease, that is, of the affection of the vital force,** must be the principal, or the sole means, whereby the disease can make known what remedy it requires.... thus, in a word, the totality of the symptoms must be the principal, indeed the only thing the physician has to take note of in every case of disease and to remove by means of his art, in order that the disease shall be cured and transformed into health.

Aph. 8 : It is not conveivable... that after removal of all the symptoms of the disease and of the entire collection of the perceptile phenomena, there should or could remain anything else besides health...

Aph. 9 : In the healthy condition of man, the spiritual vital force (autocracy), the dynamis that animates the material body (organism), rules with unbounded sway, and retains all the parts of the organism in admirable harmonious, vital operation as regards both sensations and functions, so that our indwelling reason-gifted mind can freely employ this living, healthy instrument for the higher purposes of our existence.

Aph. 11 : When a person falls ill, it is only this spiritual, self-acting (automatic) vital force, everywhere present in the organism, that is primarily deranged by the dynamic influence upon it of a morbific agent inimical to life.....

Aph. 12 : It is the morbidly affected vital energy alone that produces disease... the disappearance under treatment of all the morbid phenomena ... necessarily implies the restoration of the integrity of the vital force, and therefore, the recovered health of the whole organism.

Aph. 15 : The dynamis (vital force) that animates our body in the invisible interior is not conceivable without the organism; consequently the two together (the vital force in the interior and the toality of the outwardly cognisable symptoms produced by it in the organism, representing the existing malady) constitute a whole, a unity, although in thought our mind separates this unity into two distinct conceptions for the sake of easy comprehension.

Aph. 16 : ..... It is only by their dynamic action on the vital force that remedies are able to re-establish and do actually re-establish health and vital harmony....

Aph. 19 : It is evident that medicines could never cure disease if they did not possesss the power of altering man's state of health....; indeed their curative power must be owing solely to this power they possess of altering man's state of health.

Aph. 21 : Therefore, we have only to rely on the morbid phenomena which the medicines produce in the healthy body as the sole possible revelation of their indwelling curative power, in order to learn what disease-producing power, and at the same time what disease-curinng power, each inndividual medicine possesses.

Aph.25 : .... Pure experience, the sole and infallible oracle of the healing art, teaches us that... that medicine which has demonstrated its power of producing the greatest number of symptoms similar to those observable in the case of disease under treatment, does also, in doses of suitable potency and attentuation, rapidly, radically and permanently remove the totality of the symptoms of this morbid state.... that all medicines cure, without exception, those diseases whose symptoms most nearly resemble their own, and leave none of them uncured.

Aphs. 83 to 104 deal with Taking the Case (beyond the scope of this book).

Aph. 105 to 117 deal with the need for "proving" medicines on healthy persons, in order to observe all the morbid symptoms and alterations in the health that each of them is specially capable of developing in the healthy individual.... before we can hope to be able to find among them, and to select, suitable homoeopathic remedies for most of the natural diseases.

Aph. 108 : As has been demonstrated, all the curative

rest of the body, and should only be regarded as an inseparable part of the WHOLE.

Aphs. 196-199 : Application of medicine to the seat of the local affection might seem to affect a more rapid change, but this is QUITE INADMISSIBLE.... we shall be deceived by the semblance of a perfect cure... at least it will be difficult, if not impossible, to determine if the general disease is destroyed.

Aph. 201 : The vital force, when encumbered with a chronic disease ... adopts the plan of developinng a local malady... solely for keeping in a diseased state this part which is not indispensabble to human life. It may thereby silence the internal disease which otherwise threatens to destroy the vital organs (and to deprive the patient of life).

Aph. 208 : The physician should endeavour in repeated conversations with the patient to trace the picture of his disease as completely as possible, ... in order to be able to elucidate the MOST STRIKING AND PECULIAR (CHARACTERISTIC) SYMPTOMS, in accordance with which he selects the remedy having the greatest symptomatic resemblance...

Aph. 210 : The so-called mental diseases do not, however, constitute a class of disease sharply separated from all others, since in all other so-called corporeal diseases the condition of the disposition and mind is always altered, and in all cases of disease we are called on to cure the state of the patient's disposition is to be particularly noted, along with the totality of the symptoms, if we would trace the accurate picture of the disease... in order to treat it homoeopathically with success.

Aph. 211 : This holds good to such ann extent, that the state of the disposition of the patient often CHIEFLY DETERMINES THE SELECTION of the homoeopathic remedy, as being a DECIDEDLYCHARACTERISTIC symptom which can least of all remain concealed from the accurately observing physician.

Aph. 212 : The Creator of therapeutic agents has also had particular regard to this main feature of all diseases, the altered STATE OF THE DISPOSITION AND MIND, for there is no powerful medicinal substance in the world which does not very notably alter the state of the disposition and mind in the healthy individual who tests it, and EVERY MEDICINE DOES SO IN A DIFFERENT MANNER.

Aph. 213 : We shall never be able to cure homoeopathically, if we do not, IN EVERY CASE OF DISEASE, even in such as are acute, observe, along with the other symptoms, those relating to the change in the State of the mind and disposition, and if we do not select from among the medicines a disease force which IN ADDITION TO THE SIMILARITY OF ITS OTHER SYMPTOMS TO THOSE OF THE DISEASE, IS also capable of producing a similar **state of the disposition and mind.**

Aph.273 : In no case under treatment is it necessary and **therefore not permissible** to administer to a patient more than **one single, simple medicinal** substance at one time... It is absolutely not allowed in homoeopathy, the one true, simple and natural art of healing, to give the patient at ONE TIME two different medicinal substances.

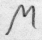